Breaking Free

Journey with God through Illness to Health

MARY HENDERSON

To John,

My anchor and my sail,

and

To Austin, Matthew, and Alisa,

Fellow adventurers, dearest treasures.

CONTENTS

Preface

At the lowest point, I was in a wheelchair and could barely feed myself or brush my teeth. Doctors labeled my illness fibromyalgia, but they couldn't offer any treatment possibilities that they knew would work. Feeling worse than I've ever felt in my life, with no hope of improvement being offered, I had to somehow pull myself up and begin the arduous, unmapped climb to the place where I find myself now—living a normal, healthy life; working full-time; exercising an hour daily; and enjoying endless possibilities.

In my work as a therapist, I now help people with life-defining illnesses similar to mine, though they may be labeled differently: lupus, migraines, chronic fatigue, depression, debilitating anxiety, diabetes, and musculoskeletal problems, to name a few. In each case, the challenge is the same: finding the path—and often the ongoing motivation—to forge ahead through a maze of alternative and conventional medical possibilities on the quest to find treatments that will lead to significant improvement, and sometimes, fullness of health.

Because I was able to do this myself against insurmountable obstacles, I'm passionate about helping others to do so as well. I invite you to travel with me in these pages as I describe my own sudden, startling health loss while living overseas, followed by my battle through the jungles of modern American medicine. My own journey included spiritual as well as medical searching. I desperately needed God's guidance and encouragement, even though struggling with the universal questions of his involvement in the suffering that now I so acutely experienced. At times, God seemed distant; at other times, he seemed refreshing and pragmatic—and in the end, I have come to experience a relationship with him that is deep and richly fulfilling.

As you journey with me, I'll guide you in creating your own dynamic battle plan for achieving greater physical health along with emotional and spiritual well-being. It may be tempting to skip over some of the exercises or Scripture contemplations, but I strongly encourage you not to do so. These are the stepping stones that will take you to greater wellness. The health of your inner world—both spiritually and emotionally—is vitally linked to your physical improvement. Don't miss out on these opportunities to reach your fullest potential. There is space provided at the end of each chapter for you to write your answers, plans, and goals in response to the material presented in that chapter.

Also, it may be helpful for you to embark upon our excursion with a friend, counselor, or small group to facilitate greater motivation and discipline in creating and following your plan. Guidelines for leading a small group can be found in Appendix 4.

There were many helpful travelers who informed, coached, and led me to wellness. I've included their writings and websites in the appendices, and I'll direct you to them throughout the coming pages. My hope and prayer is that you may achieve a far greater level of health along with a deepened, enriched relationship with God, as well as the joy and well-being that follow. Be encouraged and hopeful—God has brought you here for a purpose!

Let him who walks in the dark, who has no light,

trust in the name of the Lord

and rely on his God.

Isaiah 50:10

I know God won't give me anything I can't handle;

I just wish he didn't trust me so much.

Mother Teresa

PROLOGUE

God is Never Surprised

There is a time for everything,
And a season for every activity under heaven.
Ecclesiastes 3:1

"You always think it will happen to someone else," they say—and it's true.

You fear the unthinkable, reading your newspaper, listening to your friend. Someone's dying of cancer, a distant acquaintance is killed in an accident, the neighbor lives in a wheelchair.

But it's always someone else—until it's you, caught by surprise. And never would you have guessed the particular gift that would come for you, wrapped in its brown paper package. It's not what you had feared or imagined in your nightmare. Sometimes it's something you've never even heard of.

Ceaseless pain … loneliness … unrelenting boredom—day after day, the closest of companions. A glimpse into hell, being ripped suddenly from my husband and three children, halfway around the world—doctors had no solution, no understanding, for the constant draining pain of arms, legs, back, neck, and hands. There was no known cause, no remedy, for muscles that hurt themselves from the slightest movement and then refused to heal. Preparing a bowl of cereal or moving my eyes to look at a friend who was speaking became hazardous, causing hours, days, or weeks of unending pain.

Every movement had to be cautious, planned—or unexpectedly, the beast would pounce.

Suicide wrapped its enticing arms around me, offering comfort. Alone every day, unable to perform simple tasks or joys, far from everyone—why not escape, fly away?

All my life, I had felt, a like a multi-colored bird with endless possibilities, flying effortlessly. Now, suddenly, there was this iron cage, growing smaller each day. Former joys, my reasons for living, were now far from reach, living across expansive waters.

Alisa was only ten. She needed guidance into womanhood. And Matthew at thirteen—who would push him to his potential? Austin: after sixteen years, there were answers, wisdom, and care that only a mother could provide.

My husband John couldn't be left with so much on his own. Burden as I was, he loved me. It was amazing.

Answers, solutions, healing—they were hidden in a maze with many dead ends. Limping, crawling, I needed to work that maze, foraging pathways—surprised when help came at unexpected turns.

How did I fall from majestic heights to so low a place in just a few months? Could I ever climb again?

The black tunnel stretched ahead for miles and miles. I never meant to enter it.

For Further Thought

What hopes and dreams urge you forward to seek greater improvement in your health? Proverbs 13:12 says, "Hope deferred makes the heart sick, but a longing fulfilled is a tree of life." Let your aspirations propel and energize you to fight for your health. What goals and possibilities can you achieve as you improve?

Hopes and Dreams That I Can Achieve
With Improved Health . . .

Winter

God is our refuge and strength, an ever-present help in trouble.

Therefore we will not fear, though the earth give way

and the mountains fall into the heart of the sea.

Psalm 46:1–3

When we long for life without difficulties,

remind us that oaks grow strong in contrary winds,

and diamonds are made under pressure.

Peter Marshall (1902–1949)

CHAPTER 1

Trust His Invisible Sovereignty

A time to be born, and a time to die.
Ecclesiastes 3:2a

December 4, 1997

It was dark—a strange darkness. It was only four thirty in the afternoon, and yet clearly night had fallen.

Our plane was just touching down in Budapest, Hungary, on a bleak winter afternoon. I felt no sense of foreboding about what was to come. Just the opposite—there was only light-hearted anticipation of a new beginning, a fresh life.

The five of us were experienced adventurers, eager to explore a new country and existence. Throughout our previous eight years while living and traveling in New Zealand, we had explored remote forests, discovered hidden waterfalls, and climbed a majestic glacier. Our three children had been raised on the thrill of experiencing new cultures and couldn't wait to dive into this intriguing Eastern European country. For my husband John and me, this move was the culmination of a lifetime of training, preparation, and planning. We would live here and travel throughout eighteen countries with our work. Yet in the midst of my exhilaration was a growing "presence" I tried to ignore.

It began months before as a barely noticeable ache. I had packed up our household, preparing to move from New Zealand to Hungary, and was bending and lifting continuously. Over the weeks, my shoulders and arms started to ache and stiffen, yet we had to move by a certain date. And so I kept pushing, thinking that when the move was complete and we were in Hungary, I would rest and heal.

If only I'd known the tremendous price I would pay pushing myself to move by December, if I had known what these symptoms meant, maybe I could have avoided the darkness that would follow.

December 25, 1997

Christmas in our new country! Snow thickly blanketed the gray buildings and landscape, heightening the sense of wonder and awe in this unknown terrain. A simply decorated pine tree and several presents graced our home, but the biggest gift was being in Hungary, embarking on the new adventure.

All the presents had been opened, and John was in the kitchen, clattering pans, cooking his annual "Dad's Christmas breakfast." I reflected on the past weeks, sitting in my comfortable, cushioned chair.

We had moved into an apartment in Budapest, and all our belongings had arrived from New Zealand. Each day was filled with something exciting and new as our kids settled into their English-speaking international school and John and I began meeting our co-workers and learning about the people and responsibilities of our work here with an international Christian organization. John would oversee the training and personal development of more than seven hundred employees in Eastern Europe and Russia, traveling throughout the year. I would work with him but keep our kids as my top priority. At ten, thirteen, and sixteen, they were a lot of fun.

Waffles and bacon began to beckon from the kitchen, along with laughter from Dad and his helpers. Norman Rockwell's brush would have searched in vain for the scene's mother, though. She was in a different place, moving from a cushioned chair to a softer sofa, settling in carefully, stretching out stiff legs.

Positioning pillows under my aching neck and arms, I drifted off with the scent of sausage and eggs—out the window, through the crisp winter air, and back to the time I fell so hard in New

Zealand. Was that what this pain was about? Wooden stairs outside our bedroom had been wet from dew and were slippery; my back had taken months to fully recover. That was two years ago though, and the following summer I had trudged miles through Thailand on a mission trip, sleeping on the floor of a Buddhist village with no problem. But now, the mundane task of packing and moving from New Zealand to Budapest had started a downward cycle.

Years earlier, there had been an episode just after the birth of my second child, Matthew. We had moved from Texas to Oregon so that John could get his master's degree before we moved overseas. Matt had been a big, healthy baby, and my neck, arms, and back protested violently after lifting him for a year. It took our entire three years in Oregon to heal completely, just in time for our move to New Zealand. All the bending and lifting of that move had actually strengthened my body. So why had this move taken such a toll? Maybe it had been that fall in New Zealand.

But it was Christmas in Budapest now, and God had brought us here to accomplish something magnificent. So I ignored my body's pleas for help, following a pattern that was becoming ingrained.

The feast was ready, the table was set. John was heading for the table, where steaming waffles were piled high, surrounded by fluffy clouds of scrambled eggs. The scent of cinnamon and baked apples was irresistible. Rising carefully from the couch, I pushed away rest and reminiscing. A banquet was waiting, and I was eager to indulge.

Think back with God. When did your earliest symptoms begin?
What life events or lifestyle choices might have contributed to your current dilemma?

Think of emotional, relational, physical, nutritional, and spiritual components.
Do any of these give clues or insight into potential solutions?
Record these at the end of this chapter.

January 15, 1998

We'd been in Budapest for six weeks, blissfully exploring the ancient city and its people. Beautiful, historic bridges span the Danube as it divides the city. Old buildings, with statues carved in their faces, speak of centuries past. Exuberantly, our family embraced the multitude of new experiences and challenges: language-learning, foreign driving rules, a new school, unfamiliar money, and grocery stores with different foods and no English labels.

In stark contrast to the exciting newness of life was the continued downward spiral of my health. Though keeping up a normal pace in daily life, I avoided physical strain and the bending and lifting that aggravated my shoulders and arms. Still, everything grew worse. When my arms hung loosely down, it felt as if they were tearing from the sockets, dangling from raw nerves. The pain was intensifying, and I felt strangely cold. Normal household activities—washing, cleaning, and even writing—were almost impossible because they worsened the constant pain. My family did the chores—but writing! How I hated giving that up. A lot of my thinking, praying, and mental processing happen through writing. But even typing at the computer made my arms worse. I didn't realize it at the time, but my life was slowly being stripped of every practical, and every enjoyable, activity.

4

January 19, 1998

"Hello, Kriszta?" I tried to conceal my desperation.

Nem," came the blunt reply.

Hello, is Kriszta Bazolgyi there?" I had been given this number to reach a Hungarian physical therapist who spoke English—a rarity, yet greatly needed with our dire limitations in the Hungarian language.

The voice at the other end replied, "Nem ertem. Nem tudok Angolul."

My soul ached as I hung up. This lead was my lifeline to help. If it failed, I might drown. My arms throbbed: merely holding the phone for a minute produced pain that could last for hours. I had to find help. Trying again and again, I phoned the three numbers where Kriszta might be found. Each person spoke little or no English, but I would leave my number, not knowing if they understood. Once, I reached Kriszta's young brother, who spelled words painstakingly into the phone since I couldn't understand his accented English. With his new information, I felt that finally I had found the prized phone number where Kriszta lived. Exhausted and relieved, I heard the phone ring—but the voice that answered understood no English. I kept saying "Kriszta?" over and over, while the voice spoke back in Hungarian. I barely hung up before tears overwhelmed me. Would I ever find help for the growing agony that was taking over my body and my existence?

———————

Do you need to ask someone to help you in proactively seeking solutions?
When you don't feel well, even simple tasks like making inquiries by phone
can be exhausting and therefore counterproductive to regaining your health.

Push through your reluctance to ask for help,
and let a variety of friends or family know your specific
needs.
See if your church offers assistance.
Write down the names of a few people you can ask for help
in the space at the end of this chapter.
Let people serve God by helping you!

January 20, 1998

A sudden, stabbing pain jolted my lower back today—a sensation I hadn't experienced since falling on those stairs two years before. I was simply at a store, shopping with John, when it hit. Such pain was understandable after a hard fall. But why did it now, two years later, appear out of nowhere with such gripping force? My body was like a frightening robot, completely out of control, holding me prisoner on a whim through a dark and agonizing tunnel. I was trying to take it easy, rest, and do all the things that should cause improvement—yet my condition was deteriorating, this time in a major plunge downward.

January 21, 1998—After Midnight

"Lord, I'm begging you to heal me. I've been asking all these weeks. Now I'm begging. You can do it in an instant, with just one word. You've proven that to me in the past."

It was a desolate night in our Hungarian basement. I was trying to sleep on an extra bed that I hoped would be more comfortable. Actually, the basement room was the back half of the garage; our car filled the other half of the space. It felt odd and unsettling, and I grew frightened as I thought of stories we'd heard of thieves who followed newly purchased cars home and stole them in the night. What if someone broke in and unexpectedly found me there with the vehicle? This thought, combined with my physical misery, produced an extremely restless night.

At around two o'clock in the morning, I gave up on sleep and went

upstairs to our living room. There I knelt … paced … cried. The dam finally burst and emotions poured out. It hurt to cry so hard. My muscles might ache for days as a result, but I couldn't help it.

Suddenly, in the midst of faltering prayers, I sensed a familiar presence, there in the room with me, listening, caring. As always, present, even when not perceived; yet this was one of those longed-for moments of feeling him: a sense of quiet strength and complete attentiveness.

"You've done so many things to make it clear that you want us here in Hungary, Lord. You brought in all of our finances to make the huge move; you sold our New Zealand house quickly and enabled us to move in record time. There were so many 'signs' with your fingerprints that said, 'This is the way; walk in it' (Isaiah 30:21). So you must want me healthy and fully functional. Don't you?"

But then a thought entered my mind, gently—words spoken long ago: "Satan has asked to sift you as wheat."

The thought seemed to come out of nowhere. A still, small voice, with power.

"Sifted as wheat." I turned the words over in my mind. Jesus had said this to Peter just before his devoted follower was utterly devastated by denying three times that he even knew Jesus (Luke 22:33-62).

"Sifted as wheat." A frightening description, yet fitting.

But I wasn't like Peter, denying Jesus. Maybe this was a temptation of a different sort—a temptation to deny his goodness and love when circumstances seemed to contradict these qualities of his, to weaken in my commitment and character in the face of

7

adversity, and to turn my back, disillusioned, and pursue other things.

But I wouldn't. How could I? For so many years, his loving presence had cared for me, resonating with my spirit. We were one. A counselor and comforter was at work in the depths of my soul now. I sank into the couch, absorbed in wonder and perplexity. Beyond the icy windowpane, a lone streetlight illumined the snowy field across the road. I thought of New Zealand's warm sun, its lush greenery, and sheltering friendships. What a different reality I'd come to know.

———————————

Psalm 62:8 says, "Pour out your hearts to him, for God is our refuge."
What do you need to unload on him today?
Let him comfort you with his loving presence and concern.
Write out your thoughts to him in the space provided at the end of this chapter.

———————————

After a few hours I began to reason that perhaps now the "sifting" was over. After all, very soon after Peter's temptation, God had remarkably strengthened him to become an outstanding leader. Maybe extraordinary new things were about to begin.

I decided that John and I should write numerous friends in America and New Zealand the next day and ask them to pray for us. I prayed long and hard that night, hoping God would bring swift healing. Returning to bed after several hours, I was convinced that the downward plunge would now reverse and things would begin to improve.

For Further Thought

Write your responses on the following pages.

To strengthen your spiritual health:

In what ways does your illness threaten to pull you away from God? What will help you to resist this temptation and instead, draw near to him?

To strengthen your physical health:

Are there symptoms or aspects of your illness that you are ignoring, but that you need to be proactively addressing, searching for solutions? Check out the resources in Appendix 1 for fresh "solution" ideas.

Personal Reflections and Plans from Chapter 1

Scriptures to Contemplate

Write your thoughts about how these passages speak to you.

Psalm 46:1-3; Romans 8:26-31

He who walks with the wise grows wise.

Proverbs 13:20

In difficult and hopeless situations the

boldest plans are the safest.

Titus Livy (59 BC-17 AD)

CHAPTER 2

Seek Wise Advice

A time to plant, and a time to uproot.
Ecclesiastes 3:2b

January 23, 1998

Kriszta Banzolgyi, the Hungarian physical therapist, called. Somehow, my phone messages had made sense to someone, and they had given her my name and number. We made an appointment for a few days later.

In the meantime, an American massage therapist had been recommended who might be able to help. I had never been for a massage anywhere, being reluctant to take my clothes off and feel a stranger's hands all over me. Desperation now drove me to go where I had never dared to go before. Our appointment was the next day. Little did I know that this would be the first of hundreds of such appointments with various people around the globe; that massage therapy would bring relief and benefit, along with pain. And I would learn that pain often precedes growth and healing.

January 28, 1998

Finally, the day of my long-awaited appointment with the physical therapist arrived. Hopefully, this was God's answer to my prayers, the means through which he would work. Instant healing hadn't come yet, so maybe he wanted to work through earthly, practical means.

The drive to Kriszta Banzolgyi took thirty long minutes in difficult downtown Budapest traffic. The streets were rough and potholed. The next challenge was parking, finding a place as close as possible, so that my aching body wouldn't have to walk too far in the freezing winter air on icy pavement. Our parking place turned out to be about two blocks away from Kriszta's residence. I ended up having to "rush," hobbling painfully across a busy street.

Finally we reached a vast old concrete apartment building with Kriszta's number on it. Buzzing a button with her name, we heard a pleasant voice muffle from a worn intercom. The door was electronically unlatched from her residence, and we were told to go up two flights of concrete steps to the second floor, where Kriszta would meet us. The cold cement staircases were difficult to climb, but the promise of help at the top made turning back unthinkable.

On the second floor, an intelligent young face greeted us, and Kriszta led us through a dilapidated open-air courtyard to the door of her apartment. Once inside, we discovered that a bare, back bedroom served as Kriszta's treatment area. It contained two low beds and a couple of chairs. Kriszta had been trained in the United States and exuded confidence and competence as she took me through a thorough and impressive examination and diagnostic process without the use of technology. She had me bend and move in a succession of differing positions, noting pain, discomfort, and stiffness.

In the end, Kriszta concluded that my difficulties were not related to bones or discs, but were muscular in nature—a diagnosis that would later be confirmed in the States after thousands of dollars of MRIs and x-rays. She spent a lot of time with me, explaining specific exercises to hopefully correct the varying painful problems in my neck, shoulders, arms, upper and lower back, and legs. I wanted to burst out laughing when she had me stand in the center of the barren room in my underwear, painstakingly going through each exercise as she and John carefully watched, cheering me on or correcting each small move that I made.

It made such a pathetic picture, with my incapacitation echoed by the stark, sullen room. How in the world did I end up in this predicament, in this place? John and I left Kriszta's apartment feeling cautiously optimistic, impressed by the unusual medical world we had discovered.

———————————

"A cheerful heart is good medicine." (Proverbs 17:22) Ask God to reveal the humor in your difficult day-to-day situations and laugh with him and others.
Researchers at Loma Linda University in California have studied the effects of laughter on the immune system. Their published studies have shown that laughing lowers blood pressure, reduces stress hormones, increases muscle flexion, and boosts immune function. Laughter triggers the release of endorphins, the body's natural painkillers, and produces a general sense of well-being.
To practice, think of a difficult situation that you have been in recently, and write about it at the end of this chapter through the lens of humor. Sometimes it helps to think of your situation as if you were a stand-up comedian planning to tell it to your next audience, or to visualize it as if you were writing a sitcom. Enlist the help of a friend or family member if you need help, and you may end up laughing together more than writing.

———————————

February 7, 1998

A week had passed since my appointment with Kriszta. I tried to do the exercises, but they only aggravated my symptoms. The massage therapist was working on me twice a week. It seemed to help a little. Up until this point, I had tried to continue meeting with people and being involved in activities. I couldn't bear the thought of not serving God and people with my passion for this place. My spirit was so willing, but my flesh so uncooperative. Wisdom was dictating that I rest more. Maybe then, my body would be able to heal.

John and I discussed other possible medical options. Someone had heard of a "back doctor," but he spoke only Hungarian. Could I go to an Eastern European doctor whom I knew virtually nothing about, and couldn't even talk to? We decided that "total rest" was a more promising option for now.

February 12, 1998

I was being sucked down into a whirlpool of depression. My husband and children left our apartment each day, going out into the exciting world of people and activity. All the while, my body held me, iron-fisted, a prisoner in my home, in a foreign place, where I didn't know the language or medical system or culture. Our best try at medical help was failing.

I attempted to get exercise, taking little daily walks in my neighborhood: two walks a day, about ten minutes each, tracing the same route, going and coming. I felt so foolish, imagining faces watching from Hungarian homes as I passed: "Why does that American woman walk by here, over and over? She looks a little crazy, huddled over in the cold, limping." It was humiliating. I'd always been the picture of health and normalcy. Now I was a sickly, decrepit invalid. How did this happen?

February 19, 1998—Journal entry

"I'm going downhill daily, walking always with a limp now. Mere talking hurts muscles in my neck. Before, I used to sing throughout the house, but now it hurts too much. I can hardly write, tilt my head down to read, or hold a book. Everything enjoyable hurts.

Are you even there, Lord? Can you really be there, and love me, letting your child endure this? I thought you were going to heal me. I keep getting worse, no matter what I do. Is this really what you want for someone you love? I couldn't stand by and allow my daughter to go through this. Why do you?

I'm a total shut-in now. I can't go anywhere, do anything. You seem so far. You, my dearest companion in the past, always answering prayers so faithfully, even trivial ones. And now you're ignoring the biggest prayer of my life."

When God seems far away and silent, don't despair.
Some of his greatest people have felt this way, including Job,
Jeremiah, and even Jesus. Read their thoughts in Job 23: 1-17;
Lamentations 3:16-26; and Matthew 27:46.
Don't trust your negative feelings; God is with you and he
cares. Often, after we wait a while in faith, we begin to see his
purpose and plan (Psalm 27: 13, 14).

February 22, 1998

I wrote in my journal: "Thoughts of suicide gnaw at the edges of my consciousness: 'It's awful for Austin, Matthew, and Alisa to see you in this despicable state. Wouldn't it be better if they didn't have to experience a mother like you? You could be free from this pain and your unknown, depressing future."

My arm and shoulder ached, useless for days after writing that journal entry for those few minutes. I wouldn't indulge in writing again for a very, very long time.

19

February 26, 1998

John was leaving for his Hungarian language lesson this Monday morning when he saw me and stopped. For a long time, I had tried to be cheerful as everyone was leaving for the day. There was no need to pull them down from the new, exciting life they were venturing into. But I couldn't coerce my countenance any more. The despair was overpowering.

He simply said, "Would you like for me to just stay home this morning?" My eyes burned with the sudden rush of tears. The thought of him staying home, just being with me, was such a welcome reprieve from the loneliness. My tears spoke loudly to John. I didn't cry often.

That morning was a major turning point. We spent a long time looking at our situation, realizing how desperate it had become: I was a shut-in, in an unfamiliar country, my physical condition deteriorating. We had gradually become used to our circumstances, lulled into a certain acceptance of them. Suddenly we thought, "What are we doing? We've got to get help!"

John called an American doctor in Budapest, and as he explained our situation, the doctor responded emphatically that I needed to get an accurate diagnosis, including an MRI, which wasn't available in Hungary. He strongly urged that I return to the States to get a correct diagnosis and treatment plan. We had not even considered this. During our previous eight years overseas in New Zealand, we had overcome medical obstacles without returning to America. But now, this appeared to be the only light beckoning from a long and dark tunnel.

That same morning, we found ourselves contacting a doctor friend in Texas, asking for his help and input. His advice concurred with the doctor in Budapest, and he offered to set up an appointment with a neurosurgeon (his recommendation based upon the details I described) to fully investigate my symptoms. By the end of the day, the appointment was made and my flight was scheduled to leave in forty-eight hours for Austin, Texas, where we had family, friends, and a supportive church.

Equal portions of hope and fear occupied my mind, and yet there seemed no other logical option.

Looking back, the hand of God was guiding our conversations and plans that day. He was moving, though very differently than we had expected.

February 28, 1998

There are days that come and go unnoticed; and there are days that never leave you.

I boarded a plane alone, in a wheelchair, leaving my family behind in Budapest, hoping to find an answer in America. We had decided that I would go by myself. Our children had just made a major transition into a new country and school, and they were adjusting well despite my predicament. It didn't seem wise to disrupt their transition. And yet, it was hard to leave them, not knowing how long I would need to be away.

I dreaded the flight ahead. I couldn't sit for longer than fifteen minutes without having to lie down or walk: the pain in my lower back would become intolerable. How was I going to sit for over fifteen hours to get to Texas? And yet I simply had to.

It was surprising to discover that there is no special medical option on airlines for ill travelers. And a reclining seat in first-class was financially impossible. The dear American doctor in Budapest had given me some pills from his precious supply of pain-killing medication, which was hard to come by in Hungary. And so, armed with them and a special back pillow, I was taken onto the airplane in a wheelchair by a Hungarian airport official, my family standing behind watching, despondent. I wanted to turn and wave, but tears were spilling down my face, and I didn't want my children to think of their mother that way in their final view. It was bad enough that they had to see me taken away in a wheelchair.

The flight to America was a nightmare of pain, frustration, coping, and nausea. Airline officials met me at two layovers and wheeled me to my next gate, and then through customs. Somehow, I made it. I was greeted in the Austin airport by Keith, a kind man from a church that had supported us faithfully for nearly two decades. His expression upon seeing me revealed how bad I looked after the ravages of traveling. But by then, my outward appearance was the least of my concerns.

Is there a path or medical approach that you are avoiding, which might be best for you right now?
Talk it through with loved ones and professionals.
And look through Appendix 1 at the end of this book for ideas.
Write down your thoughts at the end of this chapter.

Keith quickly drove to the home where I would stay for my first six weeks in America. I was greeted there by the warmest of friends and a comfortable bed, both of which were sorely needed after that long day and in preparation for the extremely difficult day that was to follow.

For Further Thought

Write your responses on the following pages.

To strengthen your spiritual health:

How close are you to God at this stage of your journey? If you feel far from him, why is this? Write down some practical things you can do to experience God in your daily life. To grow in this area, brainstorm with a friend or church leader about possible steps for improvement. See Appendices 3 and 4 for additional suggestions.

To strengthen your emotional health:

Many people resist taking an antidepressant medication. I did, but when I finally added this to my healing regimen, I saw significant physical, along with emotional, improvement. This is because our emotional and physical states are tied together. Consult your doctor, and gratefully receive this provision if it is recommended.

Personal Reflections and Plans from Chapter 2

Scriptures to Contemplate

Write your thoughts about how these passages speak to you.
Psalm 42; Proverbs 11:14

Do not fear, for I am with you,

Do not anxiously look about you, for I am your God.

I will strengthen you, Surely I will help you,

Surely I will uphold you with my righteous right hand.

Isaiah 41:10

"When you reach the end of your rope,

tie a knot in it and hang on."

Thomas Jefferson

CHAPTER 3

Receive Thorough Testing

A time to kill.
Ecclesiastes 3:3a

March 1, 1998

There are people in life whose kindness and self-sacrifice you can never forget or repay. Arlene Fitzpatrick was such a person. Her spiritual strength, cheerful manner and skilled confidence carried me through that arduous first day in America of X-rays and MRI's.

I had known Arlene and her husband, Walt, from 20 years before when we had lived in Texas. She had been a source of mature advice and wisdom when I was younger. I was now in my 40's, and Arlene was a grandmother. When we e-mailed her and Walt from Hungary, explaining our situation, they responded quickly and affectionately, welcoming me to stay with them. I felt awed, and still do, at this couple's loving, self-sacrificing response. They didn't know how bad my condition was, or what difficulty it might mean for them. And yet they welcomed and cared for me as if I were a dear family member.

We began that difficult day with a 9 a.m. appointment for x-rays - 17 in all - capturing my back and neck from every conceivable angle. Each movement to a new position was painful. I tried to lie still on the cold x-ray table, feeling vulnerable, alone, traumatized. Afterward, it was frightening to realize that I couldn't walk to the car: the pain in my lower back was too great. While waiting for a wheelchair, I fumbled in my purse, trying to locate my insurance card for the receptionist. I remember joking with Arlene about not being able to find it, yet inwardly feeling a growing panic and despair, slightly disoriented. The previous 48 hours had been bizarre and unexpected, leaving me feeling strange and "detached". I felt that I needed to hide the deep fear and panic rising from my circumstances; people might treat me as mentally unstable, as they were unable to comprehend the utterly un-nerving months I had endured. No, I *must* appear to be holding together emotionally, I told myself.

The next several hours would be a true test of my sanity, as I endured 2 ½ agonizing hours in the chamber of an MRI unit. Before this, I didn't know what an MRI experience was like. At worst, I thought of a brief experience in something like the large chamber of a CT scan. When I left Walt and Arlene's home early that day, Walt ominously locked his gaze on me and said, "Just keep your eyes closed the whole time you're in that machine, and you'll be all right." I would later follow his advice scrupulously.

The MRI experience involves lying on a "conveyor belt" which slides the patient into a narrow chamber. You are asked beforehand if you've had previous experiences of claustrophobia which would prohibit the test being done. That question alone makes you suddenly feel claustrophobic. The patient must lie perfectly still as a variety of loud sounds are emitted within the chamber, their reverberations producing a visual image of the inner body which the technician reads. The typical MRI experience lasts about 40 minutes, and isn't traumatic for many people. My MRI, however, was to last 2 ½ hours due to the extensive images needed. The experience was particularly harrowing due to the fact that my body could not lie still for 5 minutes without intensely-increasing pain. My moment-by-moment existence these days was one of constant movement, trying to find an evasive "comfortable position" to lessen the continually rising pain. And yet, the MRI technician kept brusquely emphasizing that I *must* lie completely still. He seemed to enjoy informing me that if further testing was needed, they might have to inject dye throughout my body, and re-do the MRI's.

The pain rose unbearably over the course of the next 2 ½ hours, but I had a supernatural experience of God's presence in that chamber. As my body was initially moved into the tunnel (my eyes tightly shut following Walt's advice), I thought of God lying right there beside me, going in with me. As I heard the banging and clamor of the MRI machine, His spiritual warmth embraced me. He guided me to think of all the ways I had experienced His love from my earliest memories.

My mind ventured along trails that I'd forgotten through the years, defying the physical pain and MRI clatter. All sense of time was lost. I thought of God's gift of faithful parents: childhood fishing with Dad on a small pond in Colorado, Mom guiding me through teenage dilemmas. And then there were the miracles that could only be attributed to His hand: times money had appeared out of nowhere to meet a specific need; items that were hopelessly lost and then found or returned (wallets, money, bus tickets, even pets!) Each event had happened as a result of determined prayer. Though I had to remain completely quiet within the chamber, my spirit soared into songs of adoration toward God as I was encompassed by His affection. Hours later, when a frail body was drawn from the depths of the MRI tunnel, its unseen spirit lay shining, bathed in divine affection and tenderness.

The Apostle Paul wrote to the Philippian church
in the first century,
"Whatever is true, whatever is honorable,
whatever is right, whatever is pure,
whatever is lovely, whatever is of good repute, if there is any
excellence and if anything worthy of praise,
dwell on these things."
(Philippians 4:8)

Take time at the end of this chapter to write down at least ten
tangible ways God has demonstrated His love in your life. Your

__joy and peace will increase, despite your circumstances,__
__as you train your brain in ways like this__
to practice Paul's advice.

March 10, 1998

Several days after the x-rays and MRI, I was informed that two potentially-serious irregularities had appeared on my tests, neither of which would produce the symptoms I was experiencing. One of the irregularities suggested the possibility of a cancerous growth. The other was a "spot" dangerously located alongside my spinal cord. Further tests and consultations were required. Now, over a week later, I waited nervously in the neurosurgeon's office for the final results from all of my tests, including these new, extra findings, which were seemingly unrelated to my present agony.

Arlene had been God's anchor for my soul during the previous week of waiting and wondering. Many areas of my body continued to hurt relentlessly, with only slight movement producing greater pain. Even moving my eyes to look at someone caused my neck to hurt. Mere talking strained upper back muscles, and holding anything heavier than a slipper produced pain in my arms that would last for hours. Every 15 minutes I moved from sitting, to walking, to lying down, to sitting, etc. It was a living nightmare.

Family and friends called from across America. I longed for the solace and comfort that such conversations normally bring, but the physical strain of talking made the experience miserable. Even the peaceful escape of sleep was denied - I woke up constantly, searching for an elusive "comfortable position." And in the midst of this, I missed my husband and children terribly.

But Arlene was God's instrument of love, comfort, and care for me. She and I prayed diligently for what the MRI tests might reveal. We prayed that there would be nothing seriously wrong; that God would heal me instantly now if there *was* something. I absolutely dreaded going through any more testing - my body and emotions felt like raw nerves that wanted to be left alone.

And so, on this day, I nervously waited in the doctor's office for him to appear and reveal the findings of the MRI, X-rays, and blood and urine tests. When he finally entered the room, his words were shocking: *there was absolutely nothing abnormal revealed in any of the tests!* All my bones, disks, tissues, blood - everything was normal! Of course, I was utterly relieved – giddy with relief - though completely baffled. If everything was "normal," why did I feel so terrible?

The doctor wrote a prescription for nine physical therapy sessions, and sent me on my way.

Looking back, it's astonishing that the doctor didn't offer any specific further medical referral to determine exactly *what* could be causing the severity and extent of my symptoms. I wasn't diagnosed with anything in particular - merely sent for physical therapy after I suggested it. At this point, many people in my situation are left to grope in the dark for years, sometimes never discovering the truth about their condition. I didn't know it, but I had just embarked upon a winding, tedious journey to find out what was wrong with me, and how to treat it. Countless others had travelled this journey before, but there was no definitive map. God Himself became my guide, providing people and information as I prayed.

March 12, 1998

"Bless your heart." The pity in Scott's reaction when he first saw me communicated how pathetic I appeared to people. My family had come for a visit: my mother; my sister, Lyn; Scott, her fiancé; and David, Lyn's 13-year-old son. Everyone gathered around my reclining chair at Arlene's and stared down, their faces full of compassion.

I had grown used to my necessary "equipment": pillows propped under my arms and legs at the best angle for the moment; a heating pad to be moved around as needed; a neck wrap; a long vibrating chair pad which could "massage" different parts of my back. Then there was the stiff demeanor in which I held myself, and my strained smile. All these were new to my family, and suddenly I was self-conscious, realizing how awkward I must appear.

Yet they extended warmth and love, soothing ointments. My mother had called me every day since my arrival in the States. She lived in a small town about an hour from where I was staying. Lyn had driven three hours from her home for this day, along with Scott and David. We went to lunch at a nearby restaurant, my first outing, for reasons other than medical purposes, since I'd come back to the States. I relished this opportunity for their companionship and "entertainment." But my capacity for sitting was extremely limited and unpredictable, even with the two pillows I carried everywhere. During our meal I had to get up and walk every 15 minutes. But it was worth it just to be with them, to try to do something "fun." Their support and affection far exceeded the price I paid physically.

This was the first of many loving times we would have in the months ahead. Strong bridges and bonding resulted, which had weakened during my 20 years of living far away. It was a jewel I treasured in the wasteland. <u>It was God's gift in the darkness.</u>

March 13, 1998

What a mistake my first physical therapist was! I sensed from the beginning moments of our one-and-a-half-hour appointment that this was *not* going to work.

She had come highly recommended: I guess some people like a drill-sergeant approach which ignores the patient's input. I told her what I had learned from previous experience with exercise, and that my body needed massage and gentle, cautious movement. But this boisterous, overly-confident woman wouldn't listen, putting me through her paces of exercise and overbearing instruction. I tried to trust her and not listen to the voice within me that screamed in warning. But ignoring my own good sense meant spending *days* recovering from the damaging effects of her exercises and methods. It was the first in a series of lessons that taught me to trust my own good judgement, even when it flew in the face of so-called "medical expertise."

How skilled are you at being assertive?
When you are sick, it's easy to inadvertently play a "victim"
role,
going along with things that don't seem right, not speaking
up when you want to.
Assertiveness can be described as "speaking the truth in love"
(Ephesians 4:15),
stating your opinion respectfully, avoiding the other opposite
ends of the spectrum:
passivity or aggression. If you need to learn assertiveness,
ask an assertive friend to accompany you to medical
appointments in order to model this skill
and encourage you to practice it.

March 14, 1998

"When are you coming back?" It was the sweet voice of my daughter, Alisa, on the phone from Hungary.

"I don't know, love. They're still trying to find out how to help me."

"I miss you so much, Mama."

My throat tightened. I didn't want to cry and distress her more. "I miss you too," came out in a raspy voice.

"Dad's right here next to me. He wants to say hi."

John's cheerful voice came suddenly. "Well hello there! We all miss you so much. When are you coming back?" He was so upbeat, far away, so unaware. But this was good. I didn't want to pull them down. What good would come from making them miserable?

"I don't know. Someone has advised me to see a rheumatologist. But the soonest he can squeeze me in is about a week. Maybe we'll know more then."

"A week! Wow. We thought you'd be coming back by then."

"I know, I know. But his next opening after that is in two months, so I feel blessed to be getting in *this* soon."

Our communications these past two weeks had been frequent, through phone calls and e-mail. I longed to hear from them, but it always left me so sad.

And now, my return date to Hungary appeared to lurk distantly on a far-away horizon, elusive and unknown. My family, as yet, was not realizing this.

March 15, 1998

I looked like a crazy person if anyone was watching. I was at it again: walking down the hall, out the door, circling Arlene's backyard pool, back in the house, down the hall, repeating the circuit again.

Green tufts of spring grass, early flowers in yellow and white, sunny warm air - all greeted me during each brief encircling of the pool, before I ducked back in for the air-conditioned trek through the house, then out again.

It was part of my daily regimen, exercising in the only way

possible, as I needed a totally flat surface. I increased my steps daily, and was up to about 12 minutes' total walking time.

Today was another Sunday with Arlene and Walt at church. I longed to go, to be with people and music and worship, but wasn't well enough. If only I could break free from this "house arrest" to walk the gently-sloping streets just outside the front door. But the slightest incline aggravated my back terribly. Spring's glory reveled out there, with fresh grass and blooms, warmth and light. Frustrated, I again circled the pool, crying out to God for complete healing, for a miracle He was so capable of granting in the blink of an eye. It was sinking in, though - this wasn't His plan.

I was coming to realize that, among other things, this was a test. Would I trust God in the darkness, when I didn't understand? Did I really believe Him to be loving and kind and in control over all? I had seen so much evidence in my life that this was true, despite my current circumstances. My mind wandered back to previous years of studying, earnestly examining the Bible, and cross-examining it as a critic. I had done my homework, reading arguments from both sides. The evidence was logical and solid in favor of the loving, personal God of the Bible.

Then there were scores of answered prayers throughout the years. So would I now continue to love and embrace Him, trusting His plan for my life? Would I pursue Him for who He is, not merely for what He gives or does? Would I relinquish my own ideas and hopes and dreams for the future, like Abraham with Isaac, laying them on the altar? I knew that my answers to these questions would make me either better or bitter.

I had read that peace comes from the ability to say "Whatever, Lord." To accept whatever His loving hand desired for my life, trusting in the integrity of His character, that there was a plan which I couldn't perceive from my limited perspective.

"Alright, Lord, yes...YES." I knit my heart firmly to His, no matter what His chosen outcome. I had come to know Him too well to do anything less. This was His will for me, whatever the future held. And I *so* wanted to follow His will - to follow Him -

above all else. Previous journeys had taught me that this alone was the way to abundant life, whatever the circumstances, whatever my emotions.

I lowered myself slowly into a cushioned deck chair. Its seat was pleasantly warm from the morning sun. A daffodil rested its head on a large rock at the pool's edge, wilting a bit from the heat of the day. Had that rock always been there? I'd passed it many times on my circuitous route, not noticing its multicolored surface and unusual shape. How many daffodils had come and gone throughout its enduring presence? My gaze wandered to a dragonfly just dipping to touch the pool's surface before flying away over the fence. I needed to get up, to walk the last part of today's journey. But that rock drew my attention again, and I decided to rest a bit longer, alongside the daffodil.

For Further Thought

Write your responses on the following pages.

To strengthen your emotional health:

Psychologist Dr. Martin Seligman has conducted research demonstrating that even in difficult circumstances, a person can achieve greater happiness: feel more satisfied, be more engaged with life, find more meaning, have higher hopes, laugh and smile more. In his writings, Dr. Seligman provides a variety of exercises that train the brain to experience life with a positive outlook, experiencing more happiness, despite life's difficulty. For example, one of these exercises, "3 Blessings," involves ending each day by thinking of three positive experiences from that day, and savoring them: a beautiful flower or sunset, kind words spoken by someone, an accomplishment. This will help you to form the habit of noticing and savoring the positive as a way of life. Try the "3 Blessings" exercise now, writing your thoughts on the next page. You can find more practical exercises for increasing your joy and well-being at www.happier.com.

Personal Reflections and Plans from Chapter Three

Scriptures to Contemplate

Write your thoughts about how these passages speak to you.
Isaiah 41:10; Psalm 139: 11-18

Spring

I will instruct you and teach you

in the way which you should go;

I will counsel you with My eye upon you.

Do not be as the horse or as the mule

which have no understanding,

Whose trappings include bit and bridle

to hold them in check,

Otherwise they will not come near to you.

Psalm 32:8, 9

"Insanity is doing the same thing, over and over again,

but expecting different results."

Rita Mae Brown, 1983

CHAPTER 4

Listen for God's Guidance

A time to heal.
Ecclesiastes 3:3a

March 16, 1998

I first heard the strange word from a friend. Several others wrote or e-mailed, suggesting the same word as my possible diagnosis. *Fibromyalgia.* I actually scoffed at the suggestion that I might have such a strange-sounding disorder. I'd never even heard of it! And yet, much of the description was accurate: unexplained pain covering various areas of my body, aggravated by movement. This was my only symptom, while there were many others associated with fibromyalgia: headaches, irritable stomach, and fatigue.

I'd been in America for two weeks, and had expected to be ready to return to Hungary, all patched up by America's medical resources. Instead, my condition was worse than ever, with no diagnosis or treatment plan. Phone calls, mail, and e-mails had come in from people all across America, mostly from friends, but some from people who had heard of my plight and were offering possible solutions. As part of our work, we sent out a monthly newsletter, so word of my situation spread quickly to hundreds of people across the country.

It was touching, this vast, caring response to my difficulties. And yet, I was weary and overwhelmed by the multitude of varying medical advice being offered, and uncertain of which option to follow. There were numerous traditional as well as non-traditional treatment possibilities. I wanted to scream, "Too many voices! Too many choices!" I prayed to hear God's "still, small voice" amidst the clamor. In response, His firm grasp navigated my course through difficult waters, though I couldn't see it while the storm raged.

March 17, 1999

"These people are all kooks and wackos!" I was talking on the phone to my friend Sally in California.

"What do you mean?"

"So many people are contacting me with advice for my condition. So many are offering kooky, 'alternative medicine' approaches."

"Like what?"

"Stuff I've never heard of, maybe because I've lived outside of this country for so long. Things like 'detoxification,' and 'free-radicals,' and all kinds of potions and elixirs and herbs I should be taking. I'm actually drinking clam juice and a nasty herbal drink twice a day!"

Sally thought for a minute. "Maybe these kinds of unknown medical quandaries make people willing to try wacky things."

"Well, *I* certainly feel wacky, but I can't tell who is crazy and who I should listen to. Some of the people giving me 'alternative' advice seem like intelligent people."

"What have you learned from your medical doctor?"

"I've only seen a neurosurgeon, and he's tested me thoroughly, finding nothing. But I have an appointment with a rheumatologist - the medical specialist for something called 'fibromyalgia.' I'm hoping he'll have the answers." I was so blindly trusting then, so naïve.

"Pray for me, Sally, to have God's wisdom and guidance to find out what is wrong and how to get better."

"I already am, Mary. Constantly. But in the meantime, keep on drinking that clam juice."

March 24, 1998

His manner was so confident, so superior, so all-knowing. And I was so needy, so desperate. I had been warned not to trust him completely. But I wanted to believe his message - that he had all the answers. How was I to know that he would lead me down a garden path to nowhere, as many of his kind had done to others like me before?

The rheumatologist: my first appointment with him involved more tests, questions, answers. My next appointment yielded his official verdict, "fibromyalgia": a condition causing pain in the muscles and fibrous connective tissues, affecting at least 4 million people in the U.S. It is sometimes described as "arthritis of the muscles," though it's not truly a form of arthritis. I would learn that fibromyalgia is a mysterious condition, with no known cause or cure.

This doctor's diagnosis came accompanied by prescribed medication for pain, sleeping, and inflammation. In subsequent visits, he was to become my "supplier," handing out different drugs to mask symptoms - brushing aside information I would research regarding nutritional treatments or other natural approaches. His medical school hadn't taught them, so why should he give them a second thought?

I have known many outstanding, effective, and trustworthy doctors in my life - but this experience taught me that there are those who are not, regardless of how prestigious their credentials appear. My experience has been echoed by a great many fibromyalgia patients I have encountered. If only these medical doctors would admit how little they know of our condition, and be open to exploring other approaches. Their proud, all-knowing attitude allows trusting patients to continue suffering, when alternative methods should be investigated. And I was to continue with this physician for months, until the appointment came where my growing uneasiness and his arrogant, illogical comments propelled me to break free.

How do you know when to try—or keep trying—a recommended medical approach? Along the path to healing from a non-responsive illness, there are countless individuals and approaches claiming to offer significant improvement. I learned the hard way to not blindly follow any person or approach just because they present with confidence or seem convincing.

Do your reading and research, and talk it over with others who can help you to think objectively. A treatment philosophy that I have found helpful was presented by one of my doctors, an MD who utilizes many integrative/alternative treatments along with traditional medicine. He said that he'd seen hundreds of patients with chronic illness, and for each one of them, it was often a different combination of treatments that brought improvement. What works well for one person may not have any effect on another. The approach he recommended, therefore, was to work through a list of treatments that have worked well for many patients with your illness, and discover which ones cause you to improve.

A competent doctor who utilizes both traditional and alternative methods can be extremely helpful. You can also discover treatment options that have worked for your particular illness through internet research, as well as at your bookstore or library.

In Appendix 1, I've included some books and approaches that may help to guide you.

March 30, 1998

A doll and a thumb: answers to prayer. Unlikely but effective guides to start my journey out of darkness.

I gave in to tears that morning, as usual not wanting to get up. Why get up? What was there to look forward to in a day filled with pain, boredom, and loneliness? Only the endless shifting of positions in an unfulfilled quest to find relief from pain.

"What should I do, Lord? How can I get better? Where can I find a glimmer of improvement for this body, my prison? Nothing is working. I'm taking medications, vitamins, minerals, natural elixirs, herbal treatments. The physical therapist is making me worse. Show me what to do."

I carefully rolled onto my side, repositioning pillows, pulling against the rumpled white sheets that enclosed me. Through the closed curtains I saw leafy shadows playing in the morning breeze. As the lilt of their rhythm caused me to relax a little, soft thoughts began trickling into my mind: "What if you made a little doll that you treasured and enjoyed. You could wind her up, and she could move around freely. But what if day after day, she ran herself into a wall, damaging herself, never learning? And yet, she'd complain, 'I don't understand this. Why can't I walk and move normally like I used to? What's wrong with me?'"

"Mary, you are like that doll - My child, that I created, and I delight in you. Yet daily, you fuel your body with harmful things, and deprive yourself of what you need. You poison yourself with sugar and junk food, then starve yourself of healthful nutrition, chasing a god who won't satisfy."

The clean white pillowcase was cool against my hot cheek. Since childhood, food had been both friend and enemy. Comfort and curse. I'd become addicted to foods with sugar, avoiding weight gain by limiting healthier choices.

The gentle, reproving thoughts continued - like a shepherd coaxing a wayward sheep. "You're ruining yourself. In the same way that an alcoholic eliminates alcohol, you need to stop sugar.

Replace it with healthy food, created to make your body thrive."

I lay in bed, overwhelmed by my lack of self-control when it came to sugar. I had tried to limit or eliminate it a few times in the past, but there was an inescapable entrapment. I *had* to have it daily, even though I knew it wasn't good for me. My other food choices weren't all that great either.

I finally dragged myself out of bed and the day proceeded, with these thoughts crowding to the back of my mind. When afternoon came, I listlessly started an audio recording that had been recommended by a fellow fibromyalgia-sufferer. It was one of many materials in the growing pile of resources people were mailing. It quickly had my full attention.

"Your doctor will prescribe many various medications, but don't place your trust in these for healing. Your body was created with a marvelous capacity to heal itself if supplied with the food substances it requires for maximum efficiency."

"Suppose you slammed your thumb in the drawer of your desk every day. And yet, you wondered, 'Why doesn't my thumb feel good? Why doesn't my thumb work the way it used to?' And yet, daily, you continued to slam your thumb in the drawer."

"That is precisely what many people are doing to their bodies, through what they put into them under the name of 'food.' Their bodies are being 'slammed' with foods lacking the nutritional qualities that bodies need to thrive. In fact, many foods being consumed actually cause damage. And yet, people scratch their heads, having a variety of ailments, saying, 'Why don't I feel good? Why doesn't my body work as it should?'"

When the tape was finished, I sat in silence for a long time. The morning's bedtime message had clearly been re-stated, with a new illustration for emphasis. And yet the theme was the same: "Foolish actions cause damaging consequences, yet are repeated in stupidity."

"All right, Lord," I finally whispered meekly. "From the depths of my heart, I want to fuel this body with healthy foods. And yet, it seems a monumental task to control my sugar consumption and change my eating habits. You know I've tried before and failed. But I *must* get well. Please give me the strength."

Those who have tried to make a major lifestyle change in eating habits can appreciate the difficulty of the task. But pain is a great motivator, whether physical or emotional.

In the following months, I experienced God's strength when my will faltered. There were major struggles, especially at first. But I learned to fuel my body with healthy food. I gave up sugar, along with other damaging substances. I learned other wise eating principles. And my body rejoiced and rewarded me!

As I slid between soft sheets that night, the moon enveloped me in its glow. Against the window, deep green leaves tapped with the breeze, teasing a brown-leafed houseplant sitting on the bedside table. One was rich with life and freedom, the other sickly and dying. I fell into a deep sleep, lulled by the music of gentle tapping.

————————

In 1880, the first year they kept a record,
one in thirty people got cancer.
Today it's one out of two.
There may be many factors contributing to this increase, but
you can't help thinking of the difference in dietary intake
between the late 1800's and now, and how this information sheds
light upon contributing factors affecting chronic illness. A
century ago, the average person ate food produced on a farm,
with no fast food available,
and very little processed or "snacking" food to purchase.
Today in America, these foods make up the majority
of many peoples' diets.
In addition, farm foods were produced then without the
abundance of chemicals used today. Another interesting factor is
that, in last 40 years, we have increased sugar consumption in

the U.S. from 26 pounds to 135 lbs. of sugar per person per year!
Prior to the 1900's, the average consumption was only
5 lbs. per person per year.
Common sense tells me that human bodies
were not created to run optimally on this kind of fuel.
Learning these kinds of facts helped propel me to take drastic
action regarding my diet, and to eat foods like those from the
garden we were originally placed into as human beings. I hope
this motivates you in the same way, and since permanent dietary
changes are so hard to make, it helps to enlist assistance. There
are some excellent on-line support programs for facilitating
nutritional lifestyle changes. Do your research and
check with your trusted doctor
to be sure that the nutritional plan you choose
works well for your illness.
Please take a few minutes to write at the end of this chapter
any dietary changes
that you already know you need to make.
Also, write the next step you will take
to begin making changes,
such as reading an appropriate book, checking out a website,
or visiting a nutritionist.

April 1, 1998

"How are you doing today?" An angelic voice penetrated my misery. Another answer to prayers for guidance.

It was Erika, my new physical therapist. She listened compassionately as I recounted my physical symptoms and history. She based her treatments on my input and feedback, wedded with her skill and training.

It was an ordeal to get to her, though. Erika worked in a

hospital 40 minutes from where I was living. My church had set up a roster of drivers to bring me to her three times a week. I never knew how much pain I would have to endure to ride in each car with its different seating comfortability. The driver would drop me off at the entrance of the hospital, and I would pray to be able to make it through the front door, down a short hall, pulling heavy doors that opened into the physical therapy wing. I would hope that I could endure sitting in the waiting room until they called me for my appointment. Then I hoped I could make it into the changing room and get into a hospital gown without flaring up my muscles beyond the point of no return. Once changed, I would hobble to my little cubicle for treatment, hoping again that the therapy wouldn't flare me up for days or weeks. After my treatment, I reversed this process, hoping I wouldn't undo any good that had been done for my body. I often wished that someone would check me into a long-term medical treatment center that really knew what to do for fibromyalgia, but I didn't know if such a center existed anywhere.

Erika's methods involved various forms of massage therapy, along with heat and ultrasound treatments. Gradual improvement resulted over a couple of months, and I eased into a trusting relationship with her. But the day would come too soon when I learned that she would be gone for 3 weeks. I felt devastated at the time: my condition could go backward so quickly, and I had begun to learn how difficult it was to find someone who worked effectively with fibromyalgia. But the closing of this door would be God's hand at work leading into a whole new world of possibilities.

For Further Thought

Write your responses to this question on the following pages.

To strengthen your emotional and spiritual health:

The path of a person with chronic illness is often fraught with disappointment and discouragement, difficult news and closed doors. In the midst of this, it can be hard to notice or savor new doors that open, or fresh opportunities that occur. To help with training your brain to become aware and relish these kinds of things, think back in your life of three closed doors you encountered: times you were headed in a direction, but were stopped. Now think of a positive thing that happened as a result of each closed door. If you find that your brain is frozen in negativity, and you can't think of three such incidents, enlist the help of a good friend. And check out my book, *Retrain Your Brain for Joy*, listed in Appendix 2.

Personal Reflections and Plans from Chapter Four

Scriptures to Contemplate

Write your thoughts about how these passages speak to you.
Psalm 32:8,9; I Corinthians 6:19,20

Speaking the truth in love,

we will in all things grow up into Him who is the Head,

that is, Christ.

From him the whole body,

joined and held together by every supporting ligament,

grows and builds itself up in love,

as each part does its work.

Ephesians 4:15, 16

One word frees us of all the weight and pain of life:

That word is love.

Sophocles 406 B.C.

CHAPTER 5

Let His Body Shine

A time to tear down and a time to build.
Ecclesiastes 3:3b

April 10, 1998

"Get me out of here right now! Make them stop! I can't stand this another minute!"

It was the evening of "Good" Friday. The name mocked me. I had crawled into bed to escape, pulling the pillow over my head to suffocate tears. Happy voices drifted up through the floor below. Laughter. Singing. Unstoppable. Aggravating.

It was the joyful Easter gathering together of a dear family. Arlene and Walt's children and grandchild had come home for the holiday. Happy, healthy normalcy stood in stark contrast to my lonely, unhealthy, abnormal state. I hadn't seen it coming, or maybe I could have been prepared. The rug was pulled out unexpectedly, toppling me over a cliff, whirling downward uncontrollably.

Austin, Matthew, and Alisa. The close-knit Easter revelry downstairs made my family seem even further - somewhere out there, on another planet, unreachable. A deep, heavy blackness was closing in and I didn't have strength to fight it. I was drowning, with no one to rescue. The night swallowed me in a fitful sleep.

April 11, 1998

He sent them like white knights on gleaming horses with shining armor. Through them, God rescued me "out of deep waters. . . he brought me out into a spacious place. He rescued me because he delighted in me." (Psalm 18:16, 19 NIV)

First came Marion. In severe depression, I managed to dial her number on Saturday morning. I waited to get out of bed until the house was empty, with everyone gone for the morning.

"Marion, I'm falling apart. I'm spiralling downward and am afraid of where I'll land. I may need to be in a hospital or something."

Marion was a mature woman from church who knew my situation well. She carefully listened and asked questions, though her own house was filled with grown children and grandchildren, home for Easter.

"You need to get out of the house and away from young families for this time. You mentioned that Carol had offered to let you live with her for a while. She doesn't have young children around to remind you of your own. Call her now." Carol attended the same church and was a friend from my past, along with her husband Bob.

And so it happened that God sent his second "knight" to my rescue. Carol had just walked in her door when I called. She dropped everything and came immediately. She packed all my things and moved me out - physical tasks I was incapable of. I scrawled a note to Arlene, explaining as best I could. When I called her later, Arlene expressed her full understanding and support. I thanked her profoundly for all she and Walt had done for me.

Once again, when the bottom fell out, God's hands caught me and set me on a new path, one that would bring new and greater progress.

April 12, 1998
Gentle lyrics drifted through Carol's house that peaceful Easter morning:

This is how it seems to me - life is only therapy:
Real expensive and no guarantees.

So I lie here on the couch, with my heart hanging out -
Frozen solid with fear, like a rock in the ground.

But You move me. You give me courage I didn't know I had.
You move me. I can't go with You and stay where I am,
So You move me. (Garth Brooks)

Everyone had gone to church, and God was meeting with me in the solitude of Bob and Carol's peaceful home. The words from this song seemed written especially for me. I had been frozen with fear and depression, and God had moved me here.

I've always been refreshed and revitalized by change. Even in my current decrepit state, this was true. Fresh, pleasant surroundings renewed my weary spirit. Carol's home was creatively filled with antiques and beauty. It was God's provision and he spoke kindly through it, reassuring me that he was in control, that he loved me. As the song was conveying, he had "moved me" - to this new home, and even before that, into fibromyalgia and away from Budapest and my family. Why? I didn't know, but I rested in him.

Easter Sunday drifted peacefully by. There was a quiet dinner with Bob, Carol, and their teenage son. We reminisced about the beginning of our friendship during my university days, when they had directed a Christian organization on our campus. They had been instrumental in my life then, and were once again helping me significantly.

April 13, 1998

I was being carried along by a multitude of loving hands, with my every need joyfully anticipated and quickly met. The little church in Austin became like God's hands and feet to me. I have observed that the overwhelming generosity of God's people in time of need is unequaled in the world. It stands as compelling evidence for those who doubt that he is indeed alive and well on planet earth, offering kindness and love.

There were the countless trips - many times each week - for medical and physical therapy appointments. Becky from the church organized the roster of more than twenty women who drove me, usually over thirty minutes each way. She called often, making sure that every need was expressed and met. This continued for months.

Then there were the pants. Desse learned while driving me that I hadn't brought enough clothes from Budapest. When she picked me up from physical therapy an hour later, she came with 6 pairs of pants from a nearby store for me to try on at home, and paid for the ones that fit. When I commented on how nice her jeans looked, she made me try them on, and gave them to me the next time we were together.

There were flowers, and a phone: Patty brought beautiful roses, and saw how I was unable to hold a phone for longer than a minute without intense aching in my arm. So later that week she presented me with a gift - her own phone with a headset (these were a new thing at that time), so that my arms could rest during phone conversations.

There were many other little things. Barbara learned that I was trying a high-protein diet, and that I needed meat in several recipes. She cooked a large amount of meat that I could freeze and use for weeks. She altered and hemmed pants for me. Later, I stayed with her and she loaned me her car.

On the Monday evening after Easter, twelve leaders from the church came to gather around and pray for my healing. Some knelt at my feet, some sat, and some stood. They all rested a hand gently upon me as I sat in the middle, and their words to God on my behalf were heartfelt and touching - filled with concern and compassion as if for their own sister or mother. God was *proving* his love for me through his people in countless ways, despite my doubts about him in the midst of physical suffering. I couldn't deny his love in the face of all this.

Meanwhile, Marion - the woman I called first in my

desperate Easter depression - had spoken to these church leaders about helping me with the emotional difficulties of this crisis. They offered a solution that would end up costing them hundreds of dollars, but it was a life preserver that kept me afloat as the storm continued.

We can't make it alone in this world,
and we weren't meant to!
From its earliest inception as described in the book of Acts,
the church was meant to be a place for meeting the needs of
others and having needs met, whether those needs be
spiritual, emotional, or physical.
Have you plugged into a church,
where you are both giving and receiving?
If not, why not? Explore your thinking and the next steps
you need to take in your church involvement on the pages
at the end of this chapter.
And then, step out. You will be greatly rewarded as you both
give and receive in the body of Christ.

April 22, 1998

He sat across from me, fully-absorbed and compassionate.

"I'm an emotional mess, going through five major crises at one time. Every day I feel miserable, desperate, lonely. There's this dark blackness trying to swallow me, and I'm about to lose the battle. I've always been a fighter, but this time the attack is so strong from so many sides ...my circumstances are so bleak... "

"Mary, the challenges that you're facing would be very difficult for anyone." Steve was the life preserver provided by the church, a professional counselor, with a great deal of expertise and compassion. His office was cozy and neatly decorated, and I alternated between walking and sitting during our first one-hour appointment. My physical plight was obvious as I struggled to console aching muscles, but I was hoping he could help me with the intense emotional battle I fought daily. He spoke warmly. "Can you explain more what you mean by 'five major crises' that you're going through?"

"Well, I keep asking myself, 'Why do I feel like I'm going crazy - like I'm hanging over the edge of a cliff, barely holding on by my fingernails?' Then I see why: there are five huge weights pulling me over. Any one of them would produce major stress, but all together, they're drowning me."

I had thought this through many times during the previous weeks, trying to hold onto my sanity.

"First of all, of course there's this major health trauma I find myself in, with no clear treatment or cure. It robs me from doing everything I enjoy in life. I can't work, sing, write, walk, or even *talk* for long.

"Second, there's the fact that I was in the middle of a major international move when this happened. That alone has caused a great deal of stress.

"Then there's the minor detail that I am on a different continent from my husband and children, and don't know when we'll be together again. We're talking about letting our children finish this first semester at their new school in Hungary. Then, if needed, maybe my family can all come here in June. But that's so long to wait! I miss them terribly, and would be really struggling even if that was the only difficulty in my life right now.

"My fourth problem is that I have no permanent "home" here in Texas, but am moving from house to house every few weeks, living with nice people, but I don't know any of them really well. And it's been over a decade since I lived in Austin - I don't have any truly close friends here anymore with whom I can totally be myself or unload.

"And finally, I'm faced with giving up my life's big dream: living in Eastern Europe, being involved with the people and helping them. I arrived there at the pinnacle of my life's preparation, only to see those dreams cruelly snatched away just moments after beginning. I may never be allowed to fulfill my greatest hopes, after coming so close.

"All these things working together are too much. I'm falling apart emotionally..."

Steve's response was sensitive, caring and practical. He talked for a while, affirming the enormity of the things I was experiencing. Then, his focus changed. "You know, from what you've said, you've revealed several things that could really help you. You mentioned Sally earlier, your friend in California, who has called you many times. It sounds like her calls are always uplifting and helpful. Would she be willing to call you every three days for a while? That would give you a close friend you could count on talking to regularly."

And so, Sally called me for weeks, faithfully, every three days. She became both an anchor and a sail, with her mature faith and fun-loving personality.

Steve continued. "You need a support network during this time. Can you afford to call your close friends who now live in other places? That would provide much-needed support, encouragement, and opportunities to "unload." (In 1998, long-distance phone calls were still charged individually.)

I told him I would think about it, but wasn't sure I could finance a lot of long-distance phone calls. Little did I know that God would provide generously for this financial need the very next day.

"Steve, there's one more thing. People are *constantly* giving me unsolicited advice about what I should try for my fibromyalgia. I've received enough possible remedies and suggestions to last for 10 years if I tried them each, item-by-item. I've heard enough for now, and yet I'm forced to listen politely to constant tidbits and warnings, along with full-scale health options. It's making me really mad. I feel like screaming, *Don't give me any more advice!!*"

Steve agreed. "This is one time in your life when you *must not* be a 'people-pleaser'. You *must* do what is best for your emotional and physical health. Just tell people, 'Please don't give me any advice. I have enough things I'm trying for now.'" We talked for a while about being a "people pleaser," with its underlying motivations and consequences.

Steve's insightful perspectives and pragmatic suggestions proved very helpful. In the following weeks, we met five times, talking through a variety of issues and circumstances. His suggestions varied from spiritual changes in my thinking to practical daily actions. We talked about passages from the Bible and how they applied to my situation. I had been skeptical of counselors in the past, but it was obvious that God had gifted and trained this man to significantly help people. And I was grateful to be the beneficiary of his giftings.

April 23, 1999

"Mary, God has got a plan." She repeated these words each time she called, and this conversation was no different.

"God has got a plan. He *is* working through this." It was Margaret, my elderly friend, calling from California. Actually, she was a friend of my husband's family, and I had hardly known her before this ordeal. Margaret herself was very ill, yet she called me faithfully, regularly. Because of her illness, she understood. She was part of the "Fellowship of the Suffering" that I had joined.

"My elderly sister came to see me yesterday," Margaret quipped. "She doesn't like to come, because I'm so boring!" We laughed through tears, understanding so well this dilemma of the ill. We want visitors, but have nothing to offer. We sense our visitor's difficulty in being with us, but can't alleviate it.

"Margaret, I'm seeing a counselor here. The church is paying for it, and it's helping me so much."

"How's it helping you, honey?" Margaret's voice was accepting and grandmotherly.

"Well, Steve helps me to think through things objectively, from God's perspective. And he's so practical. Like, right now, I'm doing one of the very things he advised."

"What's that?"

"Well, Steve suggested I talk to close friends on the phone long-distance several times a week, since I don't have any established, long-time friendships here any more."

"Oh, I want to help with that! I'm sending you a check in the mail today for $500.00. That way, you can call people and talk a long time without worrying."

I was speechless. "Margaret….I don't know what to say. I don't want to let you do that."

"The Lord has given me money, and I want to use it to help you. Let me do this for Him, and you."

And so, once again, God provided through His people. He was catering to my every need, before I even asked. It was perplexing to me that He wouldn't answer my biggest need, for healing, but exorbitantly met countless smaller needs. This proved to me that He was, indeed, still actively loving me, and that He was, indeed, answering my prayer for quick healing. His answer, for now, was "no."

April 25, 1999

I could hardly believe it! She was coming! Brigitte was coming!

One of my closest friends was coming to live with me for two weeks. We would stay together in a guest house on a ranch on the outskirts of Austin. She wanted to come and care for me, drive me to my appointments, and just be with me. It was like receiving a longed-for gift on Christmas morning.

Brigitte was living in Dallas while her husband, Craig, was attending seminary there. We had worked with them during our eight years in New Zealand, and thought we'd never see each other again when we each moved to opposite parts of the world. She knew how needy I was now, and wanted to come help.

"She's bad, Craig. She's really bad," she had told her husband after one of our phone conversations. I didn't realize how acutely my misery revealed itself, even across the miles through phone lines.

Brigitte would come in a couple of weeks - another life preserver. Until then, could I keep my head above water against the constant undertow?

April 27, 1998

Darkness closed in again during the long period of waiting.

Each day crawled slowly along, feeling like a week in its passing.

Each day was another day to have to wake up...to have to get out of bed. What for? For a day filled with frustration, tedium, hurt, and isolation.

I was getting only microscopically better. I could walk for 15 minutes daily now. It was doubtful that the pills I was popping were helping at all. I could sometimes sit for 30 minutes at a time before having to walk restlessly through the house again.

My tight, painful muscles were a cruel taskmaster, always threatening to hurl me backwards from any progress I'd made. My body was a prison, limiting and punishing me.

I still couldn't hold a book to read it, or write more than one or two sentences. I couldn't stand in one place for more than five seconds without having to move. I was housebound, other than my required medical trips. Merciful friends tried to help me "get out" for a while, and I could walk in the mall or department store for five or ten minutes, careful to not stray far from the entrance, where I could quickly escape damaging pain and be driven home.

Just walking into my physical therapy appointment was still an unpredictable chore. Would I make it down the corridor, into the office, through the hallway, and into Erika's cubicle without my back tightening, stubbornly refusing treatment? And then could I make it back to the car afterward, to sit for the long drive home?

Erika, the physical therapist, kept working fervently on me three times a week, but I could tell she was perplexed by my condition. I should have been getting better, faster.

And the rheumatologist actually seemed mad at me for not improving more rapidly. I seemed to be a threat to him - I wasn't getting better under his care, so it must be *my* fault.

Each day was another day to live in someone else's home, to fit into *their* schedule and life. To have to talk politely, when inside I was screaming.

Every day I missed my sweet family. What were their moments like? Alisa was so young; she needed my nurturing and sensitivity. Matthew was on the verge of adolescence, forever leaving childhood behind. I prayed, "Lord, please don't let him cross that line while I'm gone, as they do overnight. Can I please be with him for just a little while before that happens?" Austin was 16, and needed me to help guide him through treacherous teenage waters. And how was John doing as a single father after two months in a strange, new country? He was probably so weary.

My back was killing me. I needed to get out of bed, to change positions, to move. But the day ahead was overwhelming and long.

"Why are You doing this to me, Lord? You could heal me in an instant. You are allowing all this misery. I don't understand why."

Mary, if there was any other way to accomplish what I need to, I would do it.

It was that still, small voice again. Gentle, kind, and strong.

"All things work together for good for those who love God, and are called according to His purpose." (Romans 8:28)

I pondered these thoughts and their implications. As

before, the thoughts had come out of nowhere, into my mind, into my spirit.

Carefully pushing myself to an upright position, I sat on the edge of the bed for a while. A few rays of sunlight had pushed their way through the leaves outside the window, and now formed a scattered pattern on the carpet, leading like a pathway to the closed bedroom door. And beyond that door stretched the long, unknown day.

I didn't know *what* he was "accomplishing," but I knew *him.* In all our years together, I had drunk deeply of his love and goodness. I knew that nothing happened apart from Him - not even the death of one sparrow (Matthew 10:29). And he was allowing this, in his love, for a good purpose. Like Margaret said, "God has got a plan." I could trust, and move onward through the fog. I could go through this day. He had spoken to me.

For Further Thought

Write your responses on the following pages.

To strengthen your emotional health:

When the battle becomes overwhelming, anxiety and depression rob the body of needed healing resources. In coping with your illness, are you holding in certain emotions, like fear or sadness? Hidden emotions can fester and make you worse. Make it a habit to express feelings in a journal, to a good friend, and to God, and negative feelings will begin to lose their destructive power. Begin this process by writing here about your current emotions regarding your chronic illness. Are you feeling frustrated, fearful, angry, disappointed, content? Why are you at your current place emotionally? Also, consider seeing a reliable counselor for helpful support and guidance. See Appendix 2 for counseling referrals. Then, why not contact them today!?

Personal Reflections and Plans from Chapter Five

Scriptures to Contemplate

Write your thoughts about how these passages speak to you.
Ephesians 4:15,16; Matthew 6:19-34

Behold, how good and how pleasant it is

For brothers to dwell together in unity!

Psalm 133:1

I no doubt deserved my enemies,

but I don't believe I deserved my friends.

Walt Whitman

CHAPTER 6

Proactively Seek Friends

A time to weep and a time to laugh.
Ecclesiastes 3:4a

May 1, 1998

The ranch welcomed us lightheartedly, jostling the car as we drove down its winding road. It was an oasis in the desert.

Even more inviting were the people who lived there. Warmly smiling, Spike and Gail Owen greeted Brigitte and me as we drove up to the guest house nestled in cedar trees, adjacent to their home. Beauty was everywhere: Gail's touch was evident in each detail of both houses and their landscaping. The ranch itself, with its handful of longhorn cattle, emanated the unique charm of the Texas hill country. It felt like unseen entities were conspiring to wrap me securely in a blanket of care and affection.

John and I had known Spike and Gail for many years. I had called Gail weeks before, needing her warmth and encouragement. During our conversation, she offered her guesthouse if I needed a place to stay. Brigitte's visit coincided with the house's availability in May, and so there we were.

The effects of my two weeks with Brigitte were like a long, soothing immersion in a warm bath. She and I shared a friendship of great transparency and acceptance. Brigitte anticipated and met my numerous daily needs with joy and patience. I felt comfortable trying "new" things with her, like driving for the first time in five months. My stiff muscles only allowed for three minutes at first, which gradually increased to about eight before she left.

Brigitte took me to church for the first time in months, providing the safety net of being ready to leave after five minutes if my back wouldn't cooperate with sitting. Surprisingly, I was able to stay the entire hour, standing or walking in back several times. Each afternoon we would rest, listening to soothing music. We also went to shops and restaurants, just for fun, something I hadn't done in so long. Again, I could do things with her easily, because I knew she truly wouldn't mind leaving at a moment's notice. Gail joined us for some of our outings and talks, slipping away from her four young children. The mixture of enjoyment and friendship had a healing effect, and my physical condition noticeably improved.

Brigitte and I marveled that we would be given such an opportunity as this - two weeks to enjoy each other, away from the details of normal life. It was something I could thank God for wholeheartedly, in the midst of so many difficulties. As the time approached for her departure, I would have been devastated if God had not revealed something else he had in store.

May 11, 1998

Soft grey clouds hung loosely overhead as Brigitte drove away down the dusty ranch road. But as the sun moved higher into the sky, the clouds gave way to glowing warmth and light. A playful breeze began to tickle the cedars and scrub brush, growing into a warm wind. It heralded the approach of a tumbleweed, blowing along that same road, full of life and energy: it was Sally, cheerfully arriving just a few hours after Brigitte left.

Sally, my friend from California, who had been calling faithfully every three days for weeks. She had planned a trip to visit her mother in Dallas, and decided to swing down to be with me for two weeks.

Life with Sally meant meals out every day, videos every night, and more fun in between. Her strategy was to fill our days with as much pleasure as I could take in my decrepit condition.

I longed to experience an American mall, having been overseas for so long, but I still could barely walk to more than two or three stores. Sally talked me into a wheelchair, which she playfully whisked from store to store. In one creative designer shop, we both loved an artsy shirt. Sally said, "Why don't you get it?" When I told her I couldn't spend that much, she grabbed into her purse and whipped out two $50.00 bills. Holding up one in each hand, she joyously proclaimed, "I have money!" and bought it for me. She then wheeled me through an exclusive department store, asking for perfume samples at each cosmetic counter. When I accused her of taking advantage of an invalid for material gain, she just laughed and kept going.

Back at home, Sally helped me organize into files the scores of paperwork I had accumulated - medical bills, insurance forms, and fibromyalgia information. She helped me think through future medical and personal options. We talked candidly about our lives, families, and God. Time seemed to stand still, and I could sometimes forget the predicament I was in, and what my future might hold.

But as Sally's time of departure drew near, the great "unknowns" loomed ominously ahead. Where would I stay next? Spike and Gail's guest house was full for the summer. Would I ever be well enough to return to Hungary? Should my family join me in the States? Should I turn a corner, and try some new "alternative" medical approaches for my health? There were many questions, and no simple answers. But time was passing, and some decisions had to be made.

At each stage of life, it's helpful to have a mentor/coach to help you grow to the next level, whether spiritually, emotionally, or in your health.
Mentors can be a few steps ahead of you in life, but they can also be "peer mentors" or mentors in specialized areas, like parenting, marriage, or organizational skills.
Many churches have mentoring programs, matching people

<u>with a suitable mentor.</u>
Consider a program like this, or asking someone to mentor you.
There are also life coaches you can pay to help you achieve your goals.
Write down your thoughts, desires, and goals concerning this at the end of this chapter, along with a few names of possible mentors or coaches,
either for life in general or specific areas of need.
<u>And don't forget, physical improvement is closely tied to how well we're doing in other areas of life.</u>

May 18, 1999

"I don't know, John. I don't know what to do." My husband and I were having our weekly phone conversation.

"Well, on a scale of 0-100, how would you rate your health now?" he asked.

"When I arrived in the States on March 1, I'd say I was at about a 15 in terms of my overall physical capacity. When I think about it, I was almost like a quadriplegic, with everything from my neck down practically unusable because of pain and stiffness. I'd say I'm about up to a 50 now - 50% of my total capacity."

"So can you see yourself coming back to Hungary now?"

"I want to say yes, but there's no way."

Not in the foreseeable future. The lifestyle there was too hard, especially with going through the overall adjustment to a new country and not speaking the language. I knew I would plummet even further downward with all the emotional stress.

"And there's no way to know *when* you'll be well enough to return," he continued.

"I know.....I know. You all could come over here for the summer, and maybe I'd be well enough to return when school starts in September. But what would we do with our apartment in Budapest, with all our furniture in it? How could we afford to keep it, *and* rent a place here? How would we get a car? And where would we get the money for your four plane tickets? I *hate* being the source of so much financial and emotional strain for all of us. It seems like a total waste of money and time, this whole ordeal. It would cost God a lot less of his resources if he would just heal me!"

"We'll do whatever is needed to take care of you, Mary. Don't even think about the money - let me worry about that. What do you really want us to do, what do *you* need. We'll come *now* if you need us to. I've told you that all along. I'll take the kids out of school, and we'll come."

John was an anchor I clung to in times of crisis. Even through the vastness of space that separated us, his stability gave me strength.

"No, no, don't come now. It'd be too hard on Austin, Matt and Alisa. They're just getting settled from the ordeal of the move. I want them to at least finish the semester, to have *that* bit of normalcy in all this.

"John, I've been talking to Steve, the counselor, and he's helped me to think through all this. He pointed out how much my emotional well-being with Brigitte and Sally has caused greater physical improvement. I'm realizing that moving from house to house here with different church families, as wonderful as they are, has been a strain. But mostly, being away from you and the kids takes an enormous emotional toll. I'm so unhappy without all of you - I need you so much."

"That's all you need to say then. We're coming. Will it be now, or June 11 when school gets out?"

I wanted them so badly now, but my mother's heart couldn't do that to my children, yanking them out of school.

"I want to try to hold out until June 11. Sally leaves on

May 22. That means I'll have to find a place to stay for three weeks. I want to try it."

We hung up, and a dark gloom and darkness descended, permeating everything. I was coming to the end of my capacity to live in yet another new situation. But for my kids, I wanted to try.

May 19, 1998

Sally got busy. As soon as I told her about my conversation with John, and our decision about the family coming, she started making calls for me. I so appreciated her understanding that I wasn't in any state to do all that was needed to prepare for the coming weeks. She found a place our family could stay cheaply for the summer, and set up the details. She helped me arrange the next place I would stay after she left. We bought lots of health food, so I wouldn't inconvenience my next hostess with unusual requests.

But I was tumbling, sliding off the cliff again, holding on by my fingernails. I *dreaded* the weeks of waiting for my family to arrive. These weeks with Brigitte and Sally had been an oasis, an eye in the storm. I didn't want to go back to life as it had been. And yet I had to.

And then, the night before Sally left, the bottom fell out.

May 21, 1998

"Where will I go? What will I do?"

Sally and Gail cried with me as I lay curled up on the couch. It's almost humorous looking back - the three of us wailing together. If someone had walked in, they would have thought someone had died.

I'd just learned that the living arrangements I had planned for after Sally left, had fallen through. My future already looked bleak and hopeless, and this was the final proverbial straw.

"You can stay here for a few days, until our next company

arrives," Gail offered.

Sally joined in. "I *know* there are many from the church who will want you. Let me make some calls."

"I don't want to burden anyone else. I don't want to go begging again! I don't know if I can adjust to another new situation." Sally and Gail continued to cry with me, grieving together for this whole mess I found myself in.

Before long, though, Sally quietly slipped to the phone, and began making arrangements. In no time, she had several options for me to choose from for my future "home."

We arranged that I would stay at Gail's for a couple more days, then move in with a family who had already lovingly helped me in numerous ways.

But in the meantime, I wept.

May 24, 1998

"John, I can't do it. I need you to come *now*." I said it.

I couldn't wait three long weeks. Sally had left a couple of days earlier. Her car driving away down the winding road pulled away the final remnants of spring, replaced by suffocating Texas summer heat. It hung heavily, pressing in. I was still at the guest house, and alone. My body was getting worse. I needed my family now.

"I'll call the travel agent," John said, not missing a beat.

And so it was done. Now, all I needed to do was wait for his call telling me *when*.

May 25, 1998

"I've got some good news, and some bad news."

I braced myself to hear John's next words as he called from Budapest. I had experienced enough bad news these past months. I couldn't take any more. I was a broken-down house that could be toppled by a single touch.

"The good news is that the airline *will* change our tickets to an earlier date than June 11. The *bad* news is that the only available date is June 3."

Nine days - it seemed like an eternity, especially with the prospect of once again moving in with a new family, adjusting to a new environment. Why had I allowed my hopes to rise, expecting them to come in a few days? Could I hold off the encroaching blackness that long?

Like with so many areas in my life, I had no choice.

I had to try.

For Further Thought

Write your responses on the following pages.

To strengthen your emotional and relational health:

We all need a variety of friendships in our lives: some friends provide meaningful conversation, others we enjoy with our family, others are great for a fun time. Pray for and proactively seek a variety of diverse individuals. If we expect too much from any one individual, we run the risk of exhausting them and our relationship.

Write down your list of current friends, adding potential relationships that you might seek to develop. Then write down what you can do to nurture or begin establishing supportive friendships: friendly phone calls or text messages, going for a walk together, a thoughtful note, inviting someone to do something special, inviting them for a snack or meal - the possibilities are countless!

Personal Reflections and Plans from Chapter Six

Scriptures to Contemplate

Write your thoughts about how these passages speak to you.
II Corinthians 12:7-10; Psalm 73:21-28

Summer

I would have despaired unless I had believed

that I would see the goodness of the Lord

in the land of the living.

Wait for the Lord; Be strong and let your heart take courage;

Yes, wait for the Lord.

Psalm 27: 13, 14

Life change begins when a person comes

to the unalterable conclusion

that their current course of action

is taking them somewhere they don't want to go.

George MacDonald

CHAPTER 7

Resolve Relational Tensions

A time to scatter stones, and a time to gather them.

Ecclesiastes 3:5a

June 3, 1998

Two streaks of lightning shot across the front yard.

Matthew and Alisa dashed from the car to the house into my arms.

Hugging and laughter. And thirst-quenching, refreshing joy.

Then John was there, his 6'5" frame bending, exuding gentle warmth.

Only Austin was missing. He would come in a few days after completing sophomore final exams. It was all right. I could wait. My heart was satiated for now with these three wonderful souls.

I had moved into our home for the summer earlier in the day. Or rather, Barbara had moved me in, whose endearing family I had lived with the previous week. Their home had been a peaceful sanctuary, and they, like God's angels. All day, I had waited at this new house, with my family's flight arriving at 10 p.m. I was incapable of walking the distance through the airport, and even the ordeal of the drive there and a wheelchair could have set me back a few days. So a friend went and drove them to me.

Throughout the day I had dreamed of the moment when I would first see them. I had tried to carefully plan where and how I would greet them, so that their exuberant hugs wouldn't damage me. But at that moment when lightning burst through the door, all my careful plans were lost in joy. And I was fine – body, soul, and spirit.

Extremely fine. After our long, three-month separation, all was well. For several days we let time and space hang suspended, purely enjoying each another. Why does it take a crisis to enable us to savor small things in life? The soft cheeks of our children, the music of their voices, unrushed stories in bed at the end of the day, the security of being with our lifelong companion.

We existed in an idyllic bubble for a brief island of time – a taste of what Paradise must have been like before man's terrible "choice." Then, it was time to emerge from our utopia and once again face the realities of life in this fallen world. Time to deal with imperfections and make choices.

June 9, 1998

"Why is he mad at me?" I thought. "It doesn't make sense."

John and I were in the rheumatologist's office, and the doctor wasn't pleased.

"You should be much better by now," he was saying in a distant, perturbed manner. His tone implied that somehow *I* was to blame for not getting better, faster. "I don't understand it."

"When do you think she could be well enough to return to Budapest?" John asked.

"She should have been well enough by now. In fact, there's no reason why you couldn't try returning now."

This man truly had no idea of what my daily existence was like.

"How can I return now? I can't even walk down three aisles of a grocery store, much less push a cart or put food into it. I can't drive more than 10 minutes. I can't carry anything heavier than a small book. In Budapest, I'd go back to being a shut-in. I don't speak Hungarian, so I couldn't even watch TV or listen to the radio to pass the time. There aren't any close stores or places I could escape to for a few minutes of diversion. Sitting for more than 40 minutes is unpredictable, so I can hardly even visit friends.

I would spiral downward again, losing any ground I've gained here."

The doctor was surprised by my assertive challenge. "Well, I could be wrong. Maybe you shouldn't return now."

John spoke again. "We're trying to make tentative plans for the future. We hope it won't come to this, but if Mary should need to remain in the States beyond August, our family would definitely stay here with her. But we're thinking of allowing our 16-year-old son to go back to Budapest to begin his junior year at his school there. There's a great family who's offered to let him live with them, and he wants to go. But our question is, will Mary eventually get well enough to live in Budapest? Can we send Austin back, with assurance that we could all join him in a few months? What can we expect medically for Mary's improvement?
"

"Don't send your son back ahead of you." I was surprised and perplexed by the doctor's overly-confident reply.

Looking back, I think I understand him. This doctor could not admit his inability to make me get well. It was a threat to his self-esteem. So, rather than admit his own limitations, it somehow had to be *my* fault that I wasn't getting better, not *his*. In fact, maybe I did not really *want* to get well, he might have thought. Perhaps I was staying unwell to avoid going back overseas. In that case, sending our son back would be a mistake in his mind because our family would never return to Budapest. He thought I could get well under his care if I really wanted to. This is the only rationale I could come up with to explain the doctor's strange manner toward me.

John and I left that day and never went back. With my husband's fresh objectivity, he concurred with my conclusions about this doctor. And by now, I had learned that many other fibromyalgia patients had found no improvement under their doctors either.

It was time to go shopping in the marketplace of alternative medical approaches. It seemed a scary place, like entering a maze with many dead-end choices. But perhaps there was the "pot of gold" there as well.

June 10, 1998

It was a very trying time for John and me in numerous ways.

One area was our physical relationship. To me, my body was an enemy that I was fighting to conquer as it held me prisoner. It was like a hostile entity, detached from the real me. The only physical feeling I had was pain. It hurt even to be touched lightly on my arm or leg. John and I were like a porcupine and a jellyfish trying to have a romantic encounter.

"Perhaps there's a book entitled, 'Sex and the Quadriplegic," I joked, but we weren't laughing.

I wish I could say that we found an easy answer. We faced months of frustration, each of us trying to understand and accommodate the other. I'm sure there were books written for people like us, but we didn't find them.

"For better, for worse, in sickness, and in health." That promise was created for times like these. A house built upon this foundation can stand secure, even when violent storms are unleashed upon it.

"A time to embrace, and a time to refrain." (Ecclesiastes 3:5) Both were somehow incorporated into this difficult season.

I later found out that there are books about sex
for the chronically ill or physically impaired.
A quick search on a bookselling website reveals many titles
for those who want to partake. Much that is written on this topic
is not coming from a Christian worldview,
so if that is your point of reference,
you will have to adopt a "supermarket mentality"

as you read:
take what is useful and helpful for yourself,
and leave the rest.

June 12, 1998

"Would you like for me to make a 'crazy quilt' for you?"

It was my mother, following up on one of our earlier conversations. She and I had been together often throughout these past months. Despite my feeble state, we had enjoyed various restaurants together, making up for lost time from my years of living overseas. We were developing an intimacy that I treasured, revealing our hopes, dreams, and fears to each other. I had really missed this, and now I prized it as a unique flower growing in the midst of many thorns.

And now she was offering me a crazy quilt! I had developed an affinity toward this unique, hand-sewn artistry during these months in Texas. I identified with crazy quilts. They were a patchwork of many different colors and shapes that, taken individually, would seem impossible to fit together into a united whole. But a skilled seamstress could fit these together into a rare and beautiful masterpiece, and my mother was a wonder at these things.

I was beginning to see that there was Someone else at work in this way, fitting together odd and unruly pieces of life into a meaningful masterpiece. But often this Artist's work can not be viewed in entirety during this earthly fragment of eternity. I was growing more certain of this now, and sometimes, on a clear day, I was allowed to see glimpses of the overall pattern and scheme.

Such a glimpse I was now enjoying in my relationship with my mother. Woven together because of my infirmity, our threads were joining and intertwining to display rich hues and intricate textures.

As it happened, my mother did create a masterful crazy quilt to hang in my home, a treasure to be pondered and explained to future generations. But a living masterpiece is displayed in my spirit and hers, which we enjoyed together until the moment a few years later when she finished her earthly journey. Now she is viewing the pattern in full, its design and plan as clear as a cloudless blue sky on a bright, sunlit day.

For Further Thought

Write your thoughts about the following in the space provided.

For your physical, spiritual and emotional health:

Clear, bright, pure. These are qualities we long for within and without. But with chronic illness, these often are not the typical words we'd use to describe ourselves. So how do we get there?

Detoxification – a vitally important part of achieving optimal health, physically, spiritually, and emotionally. We live in an age where toxins abound in our food, water, and environment, as well as in our media intake and relationships.

What do you need to *eliminate* from your life in these realms? Where do you see toxic elements that are poisoning you inwardly and outwardly? What do you need to *add* to purify yourself from poison that is pulling you down: a physical detoxification protocol? Fresh, pure water and foods? Counseling that will purify a problematic relationship, adding wholesomeness and health? Well-chosen reading or media input that will strengthen and fortify you? Write down your thoughts, and check the appendices for further guidance in this arena.

Personal Reflections and Plans from Chapter Seven

Scriptures to Contemplate

Write your thoughts about how this passage speaks to you.
Psalm 27

The race is not to the swift

nor the battle to the strong.

Ecclesiastes 9:11

A problem shared is a problem halved.

Author Unknown

CHAPTER 8

Try Different Approaches

A time to embrace, and a time to refrain.
Ecclesiastes 3:5b

June 15, 1998

I stood hesitantly on the threshold of the marketplace of alternative medicine today. And then I stepped over.

Okay, it wasn't a huge step – many would consider it very normal. Yet to me, it meant turning away from traditional medicine's approach to fibromyalgia and opening a Pandora's Box of new possibilities.

A friend battling cancer had recently stood on the same threshold. He told me, "You and I are new at this game, and in the middle of a crisis. We need to ask God to provide us with one reliable person who has done research and knows all the options, who can advise us on what to try at each turn. We need an experienced, knowledgeable guide through the maze of traditional and non-traditional medical options."

And so I prayed for weeks. And then I found Craig. I met him for the first time on this day.

Picture a scene from a movie, where the hero stands unassumingly on a street corner in a long dark coat. He appears normal – quite average. But as he swings in slow motion to face his enemy, he draws open his coat to reveal an arsenal of various weapons – grenades, knives, handguns, ammunition – all hang in readiness concealed by the folds of his garment. This was Craig.

The enemy was fibromyalgia, and he was equipped with many varied approaches to halt its cruel tactics.

Who was this unconventional hero? Recommended by a friend, Craig was a clinical massage therapist I turned to when Erika, my physical therapist, went on vacation for three weeks. I thought Erika's leaving would be a disaster for me, but the closing of this door forced me in a new direction. I was seeing a pattern in which seeming disaster was guided by unseen hands toward ultimate gain. Craig had worked and taught in hospital and clinical settings. It was while teaching medical students about fibromyalgia and massage that Craig realized that he himself had this condition. And so, he had spent years researching, discovering, and teaching others how to achieve freedom from its pain and limitations. A walking advertisement of his expertise, Craig was able to work at massage all day, then teach martial arts at night. Such physical exertion seemed impossible to achieve from what I knew of fibromyalgia. I was eager to learn his secrets.

I left Craig's office this first day armed with three things: 1) a list of Craig's personal recommendations for treating fibromyalgia, 2) a calendar full of massage therapy appointments, scheduled twice per week throughout the coming month, and 3) a business card to guide me into my next venture into the unknown: a specialized chiropractor, who could adjust my "occipital atlas joint."

June 18, 1998

"Yep, your head's come off," she told me matter-of-factly. "But we can get it back on."

The chiropractor was carefully examining the x-rays she had taken of my neck a few minutes before. She was a young woman in her thirties, sincere and likable. But could I believe her? Could I trust her form of medical practice? I wanted to try. Other roads had been a dead end. Even other types of chiropractic that I had tried over the years. But Craig had tried this technique, and Craig was so well.

"When your top vertebra is out of alignment, all the others that hang from it are affected – they're off-kilter," she told me, holding a large plastic spine to demonstrate. "Your skull, sitting on top of that C1

98

vertebra, sits off-balance, too. It's 'come off' the natural position. We need to re-align that top vertebra, so that over time, everything will line up again, solving your pain."

She showed me my x-rays, describing the gentle technique which would push that pesky, unseemly vertebra back into place. I agreed to the procedure, partly hopeful, partly skeptical, partly scared. This *was* my spine we were talking about.

I lay on my side, my head propped on a metal head-rest. The chiropractor carefully calculated the exact angle needed to push my top vertebra into its correct position. She then applied steady, light pressure to a precise spot on my neck. It felt gentle, as if nothing could possibly have been changed. And yet she assured me it had, after producing a further x-ray to confirm this.

"It'll take several weeks or months for all the other vertebrae to slowly move back into place. But you'll experience gradual improvement. You need to come back for check-ups over the next three months to make sure the top vertebra stays in place. And follow this list to insure that it does."

I read the list she handed me, and was dismayed to learn that I should *never* again
sleep on my stomach with my head turned to the side. This could pop my head right off again! I *loved* sleeping on my stomach. But I would do whatever it took to get well. So stomach-sleeping was forever banned! As were head rolls, and looking up with my head tilted back. I decided it was a small price if this really worked. But would I notice any immediate positive results?

A strange thing happened that night. I began to feel very hot, like everyone else in the heat of the Texas summer. For all these months, I had felt chilled while everyone else was warm. But now I felt hot and sweaty. The chiropractor later explained that moving the top vertebra had freed up nerves that had been crowded, which were now working normally, sending correct signals throughout my body.

And so, I waited in anticipation of what else might come. Would my pain cease as a result of this vertebra's correct positioning? Time would reveal the answer.

July 2, 1999

"I'm in the middle of a personal crisis and I need your help. My whole life is on hold until I can get well."

It felt strange saying such strong words to a person I'd never met, but they
were true. I was learning to assertively get straight to the point and express the severity of my circumstances. And I needed this man to help me.

I was on a roll, foraging ahead, trying new medical options that weeks ago I had only idly considered. I was pulling out the stops and investigating new things. Now, I was talking on the phone to a doctor in Houston who had been highly recommended. He taught at the University of Texas School of Medicine there.

"Dr. Mitford, I heard about you from a girl in my church. You helped her with symptoms like mine. I'm improving, but at a snail's pace. I've heard that you treat patients with natural and "alternative" methods, as well as traditional approaches. I know that your waiting list is long, but, as I've explained, I don't have time to wait. I need to see you as soon as possible."

"Well, let's see what I can do." His voice was encouraging. "Can you come to Houston next week, on Thursday?"

"It's going to be hard, but I'll find a way. I can't sit in the car now for more than 30 minutes, and lying down doesn't help, but I'll find a way – even if we have to stop constantly for me to get out and walk to relax my muscles. Thank you, Dr. Mitford, yes, I'll make it."

"Oh, and come with your hair clean. And don't dye it before then," the doctor added. "We'll do a hair test to find out what's going on in your system."

Things were getting "curiouser and curiouser" - I was like Alice tumbling down the hole, uncertain of what strange new world I was entering.

July 5, 1999

"Lord, don't I have enough to deal with? Isn't it enough that I'm miserable physically? Now John's acting distant."

It had been growing for days. Was John angry that I was sick? Had all the uncertainties of our future become too overwhelming? Had my incapacities in our physical relationship become just too much? I didn't want to talk to him about it. I felt too weak for a big, long discussion about such weighty things.

I was sitting on the back porch, stewing in the summer heat, half-praying, half- muttering to myself. "No one really has any idea of what my inner world is like each day: the *work* it takes just to make myself get out of bed, do the simplest of tasks, try to be positive."

In desperation I thought, "There should be a law that, when a person is sick, her family has to always treat her with kindness."

But people get worn down. People get tired of the drudgery and sacrifice that illness brings. People are human.

And my husband is human. But so am I. I could feel his growing irritation and withdrawal, but didn't have the inner reserves to deal with it. So I tried to ignore it and just keep going. But it was like trying to ignore a stone in your shoe – it soon becomes all you can think about.

Finally, it came out, involving a long and difficult discussion. It *was* a combination of things: the uncertain future of our plans and dreams, our lack of physical affection, the stress of our current situation. Our two lives are, after all, one life; when one suffers, we both suffer. And John needed time to work through all the ramifications of my limiting condition. It wasn't *me* that he was struggling with – it was our circumstances, and it was God. John was now having to work through the "whys" and "what ifs" that I had been forced to think through earlier on. Deep inside, we feared that we might never be able to return to Hungary, or anywhere overseas for that matter. Or worse, that I would be an invalid for a lifetime. John was having to lay on the altar all his hopes and dreams, as required by those who suffer deeply. And coming to grips with that takes time.

The primary caregivers of the chronically ill have their own uniquely difficult journey.
The ill person may get attention and support, while the caregiver is cast in the background role, often overlooked, though significantly needy and often run down. Encourage your caregiver to seek help from friends, support groups, or counseling, and acknowledge the difficult road that he is walking.
Thankfully, there are many resources available for caregivers through churches, community services, and online.

My children, too, were dealing with the loss of their mother's capabilities, and how that affected their lives. They were stuck in Texas with not much to do, in the extreme heat, not knowing their future. Their days often included drives in the hot car to my various medical appointments, sometimes being dropped off along the way at a pool or mall or other cool diversion.

But the fact remained that none of us was where we wanted to be. The result was often frustration and irritability. I found it difficult to be the source of so much unhappiness, but God comforted me with the knowledge that *He* was controlling our circumstances, and He had a plan.

And over time, the five of us were learning to rest in that fact.

July 9, 1998

"But I hate shots! Do I really have to give myself one every week?"

"Yes, in the fat on the stomach, because it hurts less there. These B-12 injections will boost your body's overall recovery."

I had made it to Houston. I was in Dr. Mitford's office. We had just completed an hour of questions and examination. The doctor had looked over my numerous records from previous examinations, and had taken urine and hair samples for further testing. I was excited and nervous.

"All these symptoms that your body is manifesting are labelled 'fibromyalgia' by current medical thinking. But we don't know for sure what these symptoms actually mean. Your previous doctors correctly tested you and eliminated things like multiple sclerosis, lupus, cancer, etc."

Until that point, I had mercifully been spared the full realization that my symptoms could have pointed to one of these frightening conditions.

The doctor continued. "I look at these symptoms and other aspects of your overall health and try to find what your body is lacking, what it is wanting, what it is telling us. We clipped small samples of your hair and will send them off to a lab. The hair tests will reveal a lot about what your body wants or doesn't want in your food, vitamins, minerals, and lifestyle. If you have taken in a surplus of certain minerals, then your body may be dumping them into your tissue, causing stiffness and pain. We'll know in about two weeks.

"Call me then, and make a phone appointment. We'll talk at that point about a specific diet and treatment plan, using a natural approach, eliminating toxins and stress, eating healthily according to your unique make-up, and exercising.

"In the meantime, give yourself these vitamin B-12 shots weekly, and take the vitamins and minerals I've listed. You may have to go for chelation therapy also, but we'll discuss that in two weeks."

Chelation therapy. That sounded ominous.

The doctor took me off a prescription for sleeping pills I had been given, recommending magnesium at bedtime as a natural sleep inducer. It worked very well. I had read previously that fibromyalgia patients should make a priority of sleeping as deeply and well as possible, because the body heals itself in the deepest stage of sleep. Sleeping comfortably, quietly, uninterrupted, and long was now a priority I'd never experienced in my previous, fast-paced lifestyle.

Leaving the doctor's office that day, I glanced into a side room where a man sat in a reclining chair, hooked up to an intravenous tube, with a yellow liquid dripping through it into one of his arms. "Cancer patient?" I thought. Little did I know that soon, I would be sitting in a similar chair, the mysterious liquid dripping into my veins as well.

July 11, 1998

"She's getting married today, and I can't be there for her."

John was listening quietly.

"She's my only sister. Lyn's been so kind to me all these months – calling every week, sending sweet notes, caring so much. When I told her why I can't come, I'm not sure she really understood. Everyone always says, 'You look great – so normal!' So when I explain my bodily predicaments to people, I don't think they can conceive of what it's really like to be trapped inside here."

My sister's wedding – the 3 hour drive to her town would be difficult enough: constantly stopping for "walking breaks," twisting and turning in my seat in the car, searching for comfort.

Watching the wedding might work, sitting in the back so I could stand when needed. But the people afterward! What would they think as I kept my head straight instead of turning to look as they spoke, sparing my neck the aggravation; or if I needed to dismiss myself to circle the parking lot on foot, trying to soothe tightening muscles. They were strangers, and I would appear so odd, so sickly. And it was wearying to constantly explain myself. Even a simple question like, "What work do you do?" was difficult to answer without leading into tiring details.

On top of all that, such a trip might set back my recovery for a few weeks, which was unthinkable. Once again, a fork in the road had presented itself, and the only option was an ugly, disappointing path. Yet an even uglier choice was gnawing at the edge of my consciousness: at this rate of improvement, there was no way my body could return to Hungary in August. I dreaded having to tell John. What would this mean for us, for our kids, for their schooling? I didn't want to think about it.

July 29, 1998

The shabby room was filled with brown reclining chairs, lining each wall. Their occupants, mostly elderly, sat placidly, hooked up to tubes that dripped fluids into their veins from hanging bags. It was a scene from science fiction, and I was joining their world.

I sat in my designated chair, and the nurse hooked me up. My arm began to ache and burn as the fluid began its entry, and the nurse slowed down the drip, commenting that this was normal. I told her that I needed a firm chair, that I wouldn't be able to sit for the required three hours. She assured me that I could walk all through the office and halls, wheeling my bag and its stand along with me. Had I really been reduced to this? What was I doing here? I was a normal person – not one of these weirdos.

I retraced mentally the path that had led here, seeking either reassurance from my logic, or the realization that I was making a terrible mistake and needed to flee this place immediately.

I was here at Dr. Mitford's recommendation. Dr. Mitford – a respected doctor who taught at a respected university medical school. A doctor who had helped two people I knew personally. A Christian man, with integrity and honesty. Okay – so I was here through a reliable recommendation.

In my follow-up phone call, Dr. Mitford had explained that the tests revealed that my blood had an excess of magnesium, calcium, and aluminum, which could be contributing to my problems. He said that the quickest way to be rid of these was chelation therapy, which involved feeding a liquid solution through the veins, cleansing them of these elements. The procedure was more commonly used for elderly patients with arteriosclerosis, to unclog their veins. I would need three treatments, each lasting three hours, and could receive them at a clinic in Austin.

So here I was. The reasons seemed valid and logical. I had read up on this treatment, and it seemed legitimate, though it was not endorsed for my condition by the American Medical Association. But what else could I do? I *had to* get well, return to normalcy. Return my *family* to normalcy. Return to Hungary. I had to try every reasonable treatment option.

"Lord, protect me from any harmful effects of this. Use it to bring healing."

And so, I sat in my brown recliner, or walked through the office, talking to other patients. One was a young woman whose sister had multiple sclerosis. This woman was undergoing chelation therapy to remove something – perhaps mercury–from her blood, which may have led to her sister's condition. For the same reason she had replaced every silver filling in her teeth with porcelain, a treatment that had also been mentioned to me. Mercury, leaking from fillings, is thought by some to contribute to fibromyalgia, as well as to multiple sclerosis.

I had joined a strange fellowship of human beings, this "Fellowship of the Suffering." It was a group that sometimes ventured into strange, uncharted territory in search of help that traditional medicine couldn't provide. Previously viewed as "wackos," I now knew these people to be fellow-sojourners on a path we were seeking to escape.

Each of us hoped, as we sat hooked up in our brown recliners, that this treatment would lead to our way out.

---

*There are many authors writing about treatment approaches
and options today.
Do your own research in bookstores and online
to discover which of these you agree with and trust.
Find a trusted doctor who incorporates
both traditional and alternative medical approaches.
Look for individuals with your particular illness
who have improved,
and find out what has helped them.
All of these sources will help you in deciding which
treatments are best for you,
rather than simply trying whatever treatment
you come across.
For me, Dave Frahm's book,
A Cancer Battle Plan Sourcebook,
proved invaluable in describing and evaluating a wide range
of alternative health treatments available for chronic illness.
The writings of Jordan S. Rubin have also been helpful
in weeding out poor options from good and best options.
These and others are listed in Appendix 1.
When you are not a medical or healthcare expert,
as I am not,
you must read and evaluate in order to make
the best choices for yourself.
And enlist the help of trusted loved ones in this process.*

July 30, 1998

Carrot and barley juice for breakfast.

Pizza with broccoli, cauliflower, and asparagus, topped by soy cheese, for lunch.

And dinner: eggplant, zucchini, and ten other vegetables in a salad.

I was a full-fledged vegetarian. Not one iota of animal product would enter my system! No cheese, milk, egg . . .nothing!

Dr. Mitford had suggested I try this plan of eating. My test results had revealed deficiencies that this would help to resolve. Dr. Mitford had stated that, basically, my system was exhausted, my reserves totally depleted. "Your adrenals are shot," he had said. This was due to a stressful lifestyle and poor nutritional choices from past years. My health had been a house of cards, built with fragility and flaws, ready to topple at the slightest pressure. The prescription? Great nutrition, vitamin and mineral supplements, continued rest and mild exercise. I never thought I could be capable of eliminating so many favorite foods from my daily life, but pain is a great motivator.

Craig, my fibromyalgia "mentor" and massage therapist, had recommended a diet with balanced portions of healthy proteins, carbohydrates, and fats. In adding vegetarianism, my protein would come from various beans, seeds and nuts, along with vegetables. I would later find out that I was moving into an eating pattern that many chronic illness patients worldwide have found helpful.

I was learning that food had played a huge role in my life, without my conscious awareness. Food provides pleasure and something to look forward to in the midst of routine daily life. And yet, my choices had greatly affected the quality of my life in a negative way. Was I willing to sacrifice momentary enjoyment for long-term benefit? A lot of people don't progress in their health problems because it's difficult to make sacrifices in this cherished aspect of life. It sounds absurd to refer to food as "cherished," but those who have tried to drastically change their diet know the truth of this word.

In the midst of everything, I *was* progressing. It was slow, but sure. I could sit, walk, and stand for longer. Little things didn't cause as much muscular aggravation – like carrying a book across a room, or turning my head. Typing at the computer was possible for 15 minutes now, though writing was still out. It was impossible to know *what* was causing improvement, because I was trying many things. But the need to recover quickly eliminated the luxury of trying things one at a time.

And so, life consisted of carrot and barley juice, vegetables, no sugar or sweeteners, massage therapy twice weekly, chiropractic check-ups, vitamins and minerals, and short walks throughout the day. Dr. Mitford also prescribed "freedom from anxiety," but the gnawing approach of August 28 was making it difficult to follow this instruction. August 28th was the first day of school for my children in Budapest, and it was four weeks away. Despite improvements, I had come to the realization that I wouldn't be well enough to return then. Normal activities still caused, and were limited by, significant pain. But what would our family do? Start the children here, at yet another new school, on another new continent? This would be their third school system in a year. How would they and John respond when I told them? A sort of denial kept them hoping and optimistic. I had to burst their bubble, sending them crashing down again, and I hated it.

I wrestled with God, but not as long as times before. I was learning.

For Further Thought

Write your responses to these questions on the following pages.

To strengthen your relational and emotional health:

One of the most difficult aspects of being chronically ill is watching our loved ones struggle and suffer as a result. Each loved one must go through their own grieving process for the losses they experience, and this often involves going through four aspects of grieving—denial, anger, yearning, and sadness—before arriving at acceptance. You can help your loved ones by opening ongoing discussion about this reality, and encouraging them to seek counseling when appropriate. Things kept hidden lose a great deal of power simply by being brought out into the light.

On the next page, write down your loved ones who are most significantly affected by your illness. Next to each name, write down any aspect of grieving they might be experiencing now: denial, anger, yearning, or sadness. Also, write down what you'd like to talk about with them regarding this. Think of how to make the conversation soothing and helpful. You might try the conversation out with a friend first. Then, pray for each person, and venture into open communication.

Along with discussion, find creative ways to keep your loved ones mindful that God is in complete control, and that He promises to "work all things together for good to those who love God, to those who are called according to His purpose." (Romans 8:28) Look for and point out the "good things" as you notice them.

Personal Plans and Reflections from Chapter Eight

Scriptures to Contemplate

Write your thoughts about how these passages speak to you.
James 1:5; Psalm 23

Autumn

By this, all men will know you are my disciples,

if you have love for one another.

John 13:35

The difficulties of life are intended to make us better, not bitter.

Mandie Ellingson

CHAPTER 9

Embrace Major Alterations

A time to search, and a time to give up.
Ecclesiastes3:6a

August 4, 1998

It was a Tuesday morning when John got the phone call from Scott in Oregon. He was the pastor of the church we had attended when we lived there almost a decade before.

"Why don't you come on up to Portland? Let us pay for a house to rent and the kids' fees at our church's school. They already know most of the students and teachers here, so it won't be as much of an adjustment for them. Stay as long as you need to."

It had only been a few days since I'd dropped the bomb on my family: I still wasn't well enough to make it in Hungary. They weren't fully expecting it, partly because of denial, and partly because people could never tell from outward appearances how bad I was feeling inside. This is true with most fibromyalgia patients. And I didn't make a habit of talking about it. There seemed to be no point in pulling others down with my miserable details. But as my family and I had discussed together the slowness of my progress, the limitations of my body, and the realities I would contend with in Hungary, they realized that we couldn't return any time soon.

Each person handled this development in their own way. There was withdrawal, sullenness, complaining... but also gentleness and prayer. We talked about Oregon, the state where we lived just before moving to New Zealand. Our church there had remained committed to us through the years and across the miles, supporting our work financially. Maybe I could continue my recovery there, where our kids could attend school in a familiar environment, instead of starting up totally new in Texas. John could work from our home, staying connected with our work in Eastern Europe through e-mails and phone calls. There was a lot of writing and preparatory work that he could also accomplish.

But finances were a major roadblock. We were still paying dearly to keep our apartment in Hungary, not knowing from month to month if we might return. Five air fares to Oregon wouldn't be cheap, and we would have to buy a car there.

In his phone call, Scott had eliminated these roadblocks, saying that the church could help with airline tickets and even locate a house they would finance, furnishing it through the church people's donations. They would find a car we could borrow.

Once again it was amazing to observe God's people at work. This was yet another confirmation of God's presence and loving care: mere human effort couldn't explain the self-denying, sacrificial generosity that we continually witnessed. I had experienced this lavishly in Texas, and now the same Spirit was at work in Oregon, beckoning us to receive all He had to offer. We felt so thankful and endeared toward all of these kind and caring people.

But going to Oregon would mean stepping away from the environment and treatment in which I had significantly improved. There were several massage therapists in Portland recommended by fibromyalgia organizations. Dr. Mitford in Houston had said that we could continue working together long-distance, even from Hungary. Craig had taught me all he knew, but his unique massage "trigger point" approach seemed to be an important part of my improvement. Could I continue to get better without it?

My body had proved itself to be fragile and unpredictable. But my children needed stability and familiarity as they began their school year. All arrows pointed to Oregon, and so, by faith, we stepped out of our comfortable boat to see if we could walk on water.

August 5, 1998

A Caribbean Cruise. A trip to Europe. Or at the very least, a weekend at the beach, just the two of us. As a newlywed, these were dreams I envisioned for my twentieth wedding anniversary. Instead, this day was celebrated hobbling around the quaint antique shops of Fredericksburg, Texas, John and the children slowly keeping to my pace. There was a sweetness in the scene we portrayed though, together looking through the thirty-something shops, stopping every half-block so I could sit and rest aching muscles. It was a cameo portrait of the sacrifice and devotion of these past months.

Tucked in the back of one store, an old quilt barely caught my eye. It was an arrangement of rectangles in varying blues and greys, accented with red threads. Looking closely, I saw that the fabrics were various swatches from a man's wool suits. I envisioned a widow taking her husband's things and making this warm remembrance of him, an echo of love, labor, and normal days.

We left the store that day with the quilt bundled under John's arm. I think its creator would be pleased to know that her work still echoes through my home today, its hues and shapes a gentle reminder of my own family's past, and the patterns and shades of love.

August 7, 1998

Out of all the unusual turns that my life had recently taken, the next development still seemed uniquely unbelievable to me. My 16-year-old son was about to board a plane and fly halfway around the world away from me, to return to school in Hungary, stopping along the way for a basketball camp in Germany. These things happened in someone else's life, not mine.

Throughout years of living overseas, John and I had been firmly committed to keeping our children in the same city with us for schooling. And yet "desperate times call for desperate measures." Austin had adjusted well to his new high school in Hungary, and wanted to begin his junior year there, living with his friend's family.

And we were planning, hoping against hope, to join him in Hungary in the coming months. But there were no guarantees. No writing on the wall insuring our future.

Looking back over his shoulder as he boarded the plane, Austin looked at me one final time with moist eyes. We didn't know when or where we would see each other next. Then he was gone.

It had been a major event, seeing Austin off at the airport. Walking the inclining corridors to his boarding gate wasn't easy. Muscles in the backs of my calves didn't want to stretch that long. I kept stopping, circling the occasional flat areas to calm my calves, before starting up the next incline. Always there was a panicked feeling just below the surface: what if I couldn't make it, and was trapped half-way there? Being carried out by John would be humiliating, as well as tremendously aggravating to my back and muscles. We could have used an airport wheelchair, but in my mind, giving in to *that* might grow into a lifestyle to be avoided at all costs. And I *needed* to see if I could do this. In just two weeks, I would need to make it through this airport, as well as a layover in Denver, en route to Oregon. The prospect loomed ahead as an overwhelming giant in my path, yet how could I ever hope to return to Hungary if I couldn't make it to Oregon?

Austin's departure felt like another "death." Another sacrifice, a "stripping away." It was hard to give up yet another thing after having been through so much. "Trust in the Lord with all your heart, and do not lean on your own understanding. In all your ways acknowledge Him, and He will make your paths straight." (Proverbs 3:5, 6) This had become the knot at the end of the rope that I steadfastly clung to.

Little did I know the magnificent work being done in Austin's life, to come to full fruition in these months without us. A work that, alone, would have made everything worth it.

August 17, 1998

"She looks like something out of a horror movie – one of those terribly disfigured little creatures that runs around, scaring everyone."

My sister Lyn was laughing, referring to the beloved doll from my childhood that I now held in my arms. Mom had brought some of my childhood "treasures" from her attic with them for their final visit before we left for Oregon. I hadn't seen these dolls in decades, since the day when I had packed them away as a young teenager.

Now, carefully lifting each one from a box, memories flooded in. For countless hours I had dreamed of being a mother, lovingly caring for these beloved "children" who had filled many happy days. Lyn's comment jarred me into the full realization of their present physical appearance: matted hair in disarray; mold here and there; glassy eyes, some turning the wrong way, some chalky with a white corrosion; a missing arm or leg. I hadn't really noticed these things, all ugliness and imperfection disregarded in my affection toward them.

"These dolls are worth a small fortune!" I laughed, thinking now of the value of antiques.

Yet how I needed the message of that moment. Echoes of God's affection resonated through my mind.

And here sat my mother and sister, embodying this theme during these difficult days. A treasured bond had formed that would not break over the miles – memories and messages etched deep into my spirit, to be brought out and cradled in years ahead, remembering these days of being loved.

August 20, 1998

It was the dreaded day. The longed-for day! The day I flew to

Oregon.

There was the long walk through Austin's airport; the hours of flight to Denver, occasionally pacing narrow aisles. Then the layover in Denver. This had been the shortest route available. Walking, sitting, swaying – anything to appease my tyrannical back muscles. Finally came the three-hour flight to Oregon. More walking, sitting, jiggling – *jiggling!*

A few weeks back, during the hot, slow-moving days in Texas, I had asked God to show me if there was something – *anything* – else I could be doing that would move along my improvement.

As I sat, trying to play cards with my family one night, my lower back ached, making it impossible to sit for more than 15 minutes without walking around the house continually to loosen it up. A thought came: *As you're sitting, lightly jiggle your legs to keep muscles from stiffening.* I started doing this, and discovered that it greatly increased my capacity to sit longer. When I rested an aching arm on the jiggling leg, the arm relaxed and felt better. From that night on, this technique helped me daily.

I smiled now, sitting on the flight to Oregon, thinking of writing a booklet to help other fibromyalgia patients, entitled *"Jiggling: A New Method of Relief from the Discomforts of Fibromyalgia."* Discovering this "technique" had been yet another of God's fingerprints in my life.

———————

Dr. Dave Frahm writes that "the human body is a 'machine' that requires use to get and remain strong. If you're not getting stronger, you're getting weaker. A day without exercise is a day in decline."

A Cancer Battle Plan Sourcebook

Even if you have to start very small, like I did, chronically ill people must begin regular exercise and increase it more and more. I started with jiggling consistently, and now I exercise 45 minutes daily! Countless sources echo the importance of exercise.

* *The National Institute on Aging: "If exercise could be packed into a pill, it would be the single most widely prescribed and beneficial medicine in the nation."*
* *Thomas Jefferson: "Walking is the best possible exercise. Habituate yourself to walk very far."*
* *Earl of Derby: "Those who do not find time for exercise will have to find time for illness."*
* *Plato: "Lack of activity destroys the good condition of every human being, while movement and methodical physical exercise save it and preserve it."*

So consult with your trusted health-care professional, and start increasing your movement today!

And now, God carried me to Oregon, depositing me and my family into the hands of loving people there. The furnished house that the church provided was a block from a large park with a pond, where my children could play and fish. Forested pathways enabled me to continue my newly-acquired capability of walking 45 minutes daily. Autumn had fully arrived in Oregon, its beauty bolstering my spirits and my recovery. Things looked wonderful.

But always inside was the haunting, the yearning: this American life wasn't where I belonged. I didn't fit in. Always, there was the longing to be back overseas, with the people there, telling them joyous, unearthly truths that would change them for eternity. Would I ever get back? Could I improve enough? These thoughts always hovered, clouding even the most magnificent Oregon autumn day.

For Further Thought

To strengthen your physical and emotional health:

There is one simple form of exercise that is easy to do, regardless of your physical incapacitation: *Breathing*. Dr. Andrew Weil, M.D. states, "If I had to limit my advice on healthier living to just one tip, it would be simply to learn how to breathe correctly." (http://www.drweil.com) Why? "The body (and the brain and nervous system in particular) thrives on abundant oxygen." (Jordan S. Rubin, Ph.D., *The Maker's Diet)* Breathing exercises improve your emotional as well as physical health. To get started, go to http://www.drweil.com/ and type in "3 Breathing Exercises" in the search box.

I learned a simple breathing exercise at a seminar that has served me well.   I call it "5 in, 5 out, for 5 minutes." Try it with me now, and notice how it relaxes you:

- Sit comfortably in your chair.
- Slowly breathe in for 5 counts, then out for 5 counts.
- Do this for 5 minutes, keeping a steady, relaxing rhythm. (I find it more relaxing to give my 5 counts the rhythm of the first line of "Row, row, row your boat.")

There are scientific explanations for how this exercise positively affects the sympathetic and parasympathetic nervous systems so that, as you do this five-minute exercise daily over time, you produce long-term physical and emotional benefits. But you can prove this yourself, as you incorporate this and a couple of other breathing exercises into your health regimen, and notice the immediate, as well as long-term, positive results.

Personal Reflections and Plans from Chapter Nine

Scriptures to Contemplate

Write your thoughts about how these passages speak to you.
II Corinthians 5:17-21; I Samuel 16:7; II Chronicles 16:9

But if any of you lacks wisdom, let him ask of God,

who gives to all generously and without reproach,

and it will be given to him.

James 1:5

Many men owe the grandeur of their lives

to their tremendous difficulties.

Charles Haddon Spurgeon (1834-1892)

CHAPTER 10

Too Many Voices

A time to keep and a time to throw away.
Ecclesiastes 3:6b

August 23, 1998

They crowded around, staring, uncertain of what to say. The brief words they spoke reflected respect, curiosity, honor. In a way, I felt like a hero, home from the battlefield.

It was our first Sunday morning at the Oregon church. John had been asked to speak at both services, retelling the ordeal of these past months and the lessons we were learning. These people had been hearing of our plight all through this time, and praying. Our story must have sounded larger-than-life: "Missionary travels to unknown territory, contracts mysterious ailment, suffers months of pain and separation from family, still bravely strives to follow God."

I hadn't expected this attention. It was flattering, and yet I didn't feel heroic. I felt stripped bare. Like a stark tree in winter, stripped of its lush summer greenery, its rich autumn glory. What remained was me, at the core of my being - outward pretense and show had fallen away. Yet I was surprised to find God's new creation shining within - simple, with the beauty of His purifying work from the past months and years. For a time, I was allowed a glimpse of the work being done in me: like when a curtain is pulled back for a moment, and bright light suddenly pierces the darkened room. For the first time, the ancient words became my own:

"But we have this treasure in jars of clay to show that this all-surpassing power is from God and not from us. We are hard-pressed on every side, but not crushed; perplexed, but not in despair; persecuted, but not abandoned; struck down, but not destroyed. We always carry around in our body the death of Jesus. So that the life of Jesus may also be revealed in our mortal body. For we who are alive are always being given over to death for Jesus' sake, so that his life may be revealed in our mortal body. So then, death is at work in us, but life is at work in you. Therefore we do not lose heart. Though outwardly we are wasting away, yet inwardly we are being renewed day by day. For our light and momentary troubles are achieving for us an eternal glory that far outweighs them all. So we fix our eyes not on what is seen, but on what is unseen. For what is seen is temporary, but what is unseen is eternal" (II Corinthians 4:7-12, 16-18).

What are your foundational goals in life? You will be frustrated if they are anything other than to glorify God by loving Him and loving people, because you were designed for these. Hardship purifies us toward these ends. And these are goals you can achieve, whatever your degree of health. Lesser, self-centered goals can result in anxiety and depression, pulling your health downward, because you were created for lofty, God-centered pursuits. You were made to operate in accordance with God's image, and He will make you more like Himself as you dedicate yourself to this. Then, you will be achieving "an eternal glory that far outweighs" all that is earthly. And you will experience the deep fulfillment of becoming who you were created to be.

September 17, 1998

"Brigitte, you know that book I'm going to write? I'm going to call it *Too Many Voices, Too Many Choices*. It'll be about wandering through the crazy maze of medical options. And now I have a new chapter to add."

"Oh no …what now?" Brigitte and I called each other often, defying the distance between Oregon and Texas.

"Actually, I've got two new additions for my story."

"Have you found something new that will help?"

"I don't know," I groaned. "But these sound promising… maybe they'll speed up my recovery." I told her about Mike, two hours away in Eugene. "He uses a technique that supposedly moves bones into place - kind of like a chiropractor - only more gently, through a massage-and-exercise sort-of combination."

"Is it helping?"

"Well, he says *so* confidently that he knows *exactly* what's wrong and what will help. I'll try him a few times, and we'll see. He's not like Craig, though. I liked how Craig admitted fallibility. He would suggest things for me to try from his extensive medical and physiological knowledge, but he didn't act like he absolutely *knew* the answer in unproven areas. That's how all medical people should be, honestly admitting there's a lot they don't know. It makes you trust them more. It actually improves their credibility."

"Yeah, but most of them don't seem to realize that. They think they have to uphold an all-knowing image. Some are probably afraid that if you think they don't know the answers, you might not keep coming back and giving them your money . . . but what's the other new thing you're trying? You said there were two."

"Rita Ree."

Brigitte burst out laughing. The name didn't inspire confidence.

"Rita Ree.....She's a chemist who lives in the hills above Eugene. I've heard from credible sources that she has seen significant progress with fibromyalgia patients, using natural dietary supplements and nutritional counseling."

Brigitte absorbed this for a moment before asking, "How is she different from all the other things you've tried or heard about?"

"I don't know - you're right, there so many "programs" and "products" out there, promising amazing results. And people who seem to be helped by them. I think I'll just try a couple more, to see if they make a difference."

"Well let me know what happens. With someone named 'Rita Ree,' the story's got to be interesting."

September 28, 1998

It was a grey, wet morning. Our car wound cautiously up the mountain road to Rita Ree's home in the dense Oregon forest. In the back seat, we carried my urine from the past 24 hours in a sterilized plastic milk container, kept cold in an ice chest. Rita would use it to determine what my body needed. It was weird, but this was only the beginning of strange things to come.

After a couple of wrong turns, our car finally pulled up to a small aging chalet, from which two barking dogs bounded. Each was as tall as my waist. A man emerged, grabbing them by their collars so that John and I could enter the house. The dogs followed us in, accepting us, but sniffing curiously. *Were John and I really going through with this? We were normal people. It was too strange, but we'd driven 2 ½ hours... We might as well see it through.*

Rita emerged. She was a pleasant, plump woman in her late fifties, with short silver hair, wearing an artsy pants outfit. She spoke with a flair, and didn't seem to fit the description in her résumé, which included a long tenure in a well-known pharmaceutical laboratory as a chemist.

After running some tests on my urine in an adjoining room, Rita took John and me to a bedroom which served as her examination area. Laying me on a bed, she proceeded with a strange technique of thumping numerous parts of my body, then feeling glands in my neck, commenting on what this told her about my spleen, liver, kidneys, etc. The confident, scientific manner in which she spoke seemed out of place with her personae, technique, and surroundings.

After questioning me about various aspects of my health and lifestyle, Rita began her dietary recommendations, which included several nutritional products that she sold.

"Try her recommendations for a month, and see if you notice improvement," had been Mike's recommendation. (Mike was the man in Eugene with the new massage/exercise/bone-moving technique I was trying.) I was submerging from the weird into the ridiculous, it seemed, but I followed his advice. Others had been helped by her, I'd been told. Desperate medical situations drive you to try things that you wouldn't in your normal, healthy state. You hope to discover the answer, the gem amidst the rubble.

When you're desperate for answers to your health dilemma, it's easy to fall into the trap of thinking that distant, far-away solutions
are somehow uniquely promising, compared to solutions within your closer range.
Just because something is in another city, state, or country doesn't mean it is more
credible, though we can inadvertently assume so.
Do your research, and avoid falling into this common trap, pursuing the "magical solution."

As I exited Rita's office later, my arms laden with a month's supply of products, Rita was hanging up her phone, exclaiming, "Okay, the chiropractor I told you about can see you today at 3:00. I'm sure your tailbone's out of place, from those two falls you mentioned. He'll fix it."

It had sounded reasonable when she explained it earlier, but now she added, "He fixed my daughter's tailbone, and it released her from memories and emotions that had hindered her for years. She cried for hours afterward, as the emotions of past events surfaced, expressed themselves, then were released. And all because her tailbone had been corrected! Oh, he's wonderful. Here's his card and address."

John and I rushed away down the mountain road, not quite sure *what* had happened, nor what we were getting ourselves into. It all seemed like an absurd scene from a movie, and yet we had Rita's products and would try her recommendations. She *was* an experienced chemist, after all. Yet somehow we felt foolish, like we'd been duped. And this chiropractor she endorsed had been also recommended by Mike. Just consulting with him couldn't hurt, could it?

September 28, 1999 - 5:00 pm

I felt cheated, violated, traumatized.

The chiropractor had been an impersonal, detached sort of person. He felt that my tailbone wasn't out of place, but my sacrum *was*. (A bone above the tailbone.) I had been handled so gently and carefully these past months by other health-care professionals, perhaps my guard was down. Perhaps I didn't explain carefully enough the fragility and severity of my condition. Maybe I didn't make that clear to him. Perhaps he thought I needed something strong. Or maybe I didn't explain well enough that my earlier neck chiropractic adjustment in June demanded that my body should not receive strong jolts or bumps.

He had laid me on his table, twisted my legs to the side,

134

and with a violent jerk, cracked every bone in my back from my waist down.

In a state of shock, I was then rolled to my stomach, where the chiropractor delivered a violent thrust between my shoulder blades, every bone from my waist to my neck screeching.

I have had other chiropractic adjustments over the years, similar in style, but none so strong and traumatizing.

In a stupor, I paid and exited, limply making my way to the car through heavy rain.

John and I were quiet for a long time during the ride home. He had witnessed the whole thing, but it had happened so quickly, he was caught off guard as much as I. Now, we shared the same thoughts, which eventually surfaced into words: *Will this cause a major setback? Is my neck adjustment from June completely undone, after doing so well for months? How could we have been so stupid to blindly go into this office and trust this guy?*

Sore, numb, and depressed, I was fearful of what the coming days would reveal in my body's aftershocks. It seemed out of the question that anything beneficial would result.

Cold, grey rain escorted us through the two-hour drive home, drizzling on us all the way into our house. For days it held us in its clammy grip.

––––––––––––––––––

If you are like many chronic illness patients, your journey has taken you into the offices of numerous healthcare professionals. It can be helpful to type a thorough explanation of your history, symptoms, and concerns, which you ask each doctor to read before treating you, as part of your intake exam. This can insure that you don't leave out important information, and it relieves you of the burden of re-telling your information over and over. Also, you can review it yourself

October 5, 1998

The sun finally peeked through. After almost a week, I felt a little better. No better than before the trauma, but no worse. God had protected me. And now, after that period of tension and fear, I found myself in a situation where relaxation and even enjoyment were beginning to seep in. I was spending the weekend at our church women's retreat, nestled in a pine-scented forest. It was a milestone I hadn't thought myself capable of, attending meetings and gatherings all day, sleeping in a rustic log cabin at night. I managed by alternating between sitting and standing in the back of the meeting room, sometimes taking little walks behind the last row of chairs. It was exhilarating to live in the world of normal people, being able to do what they did! I never thought I'd be overjoyed at the thought of being *normal*. Unique? Yes. Outstanding? Definitely. But now *normal* seemed fantastic.

I spent a couple of hours at the retreat talking with a woman who was going through a difficult personal time, experiencing a crisis with her teenage daughter. Never before had I listened with such compassion and understanding to another's difficulty. Before, I knowledgeably would have shared bits of wisdom and advice, clothed in a type of sympathy. Now, I huddled close to her, simply caring, sharing the load for a while. We both left energized, ready to take up our burdens again.

Walking in the light rain back to my cabin, I thought of recent conversations, where well-meaning souls had thrown out advice, and how lonely and empty it had left me.

There was the man who caught me after church on a bad day, and asked that dreaded question, "How are you doing?" I felt weak that morning, and couldn't muster up a courteous, dismissive answer. Sharing briefly that I wasn't doing well, it immediately became obvious that he was *not* someone to be trusted with personal vulnerability.

He promptly started into a monologue about a couple of deeply spiritual books on the subject of suffering, and lightly dismissed a book I mentioned that was currently helping me. As he droned on and on, I desperately searched for words to disentangle and escape. Finally fleeing, I vowed *never* to reveal distress so carelessly again - even on my worst of days.

Then there was "Claire." I had been invited to speak to a group, telling the events of this past year and some things I was learning. I did so honestly and encouragingly, happy that there were ways my experiences might help others.

Claire approached me afterward. "Mary, I wish I knew what to say after all you've been through."

"What really helps," I began, "is just to say, 'I'm so sorry for everything you're experiencing. It must be really hard.' Just knowing that someone cares and tries to understand means a lot." But she didn't take my cue.

"Well, I'll say that, Mary, but also, don't forget the Bible verse that tells us to trust God in everything......"

Her words marched past as I withdrew inwardly. Giving advice to someone suffering should be done very carefully, and is often a privilege reserved for those who have earned it through relationship and listening. Claire had done neither. I smiled politely and escaped as quickly as possible. Her approach had left me mad and discouraged.

Thinking about it now, safe inside my cabin in the forest, I became aware that I, too, had been guilty of this in years past, in trying to "help" others. I realized that advice offered in this way is often self-serving: it is given so that the speaker can feel good about himself, that he has accomplished something, imparted wisdom. In actual fact, he may have discouraged or even harmed the hurting.

This is where God shines as the perfect companion. When I ran to Him in distress or discouragement during these difficult days, He knew when to be a *Comforter*, and when to be a *Counselor.* (II Corinthians 1:3, 4 and John 14: 26, 27) When I said to Him, "This is too hard, Lord. Help!", He knew when to say: *I know, Mary, I know. Just rest here with Me for a while.* He knew when to be a gentle breeze (I Kings 19:11-13).

The light Oregon rain fell now, outside my cabin window. Gold autumn leaves were washing away, anticipating winter's approach. Safe inside, wrapped warmly in Jesus' presence, I was being cleansed, refreshed, enlightened.

For Further Thought

Write your responses on the following pages.

To strengthen your relational and emotional health:

Write down the names of a few people you know who are going through difficult times. Then, next to their name, write a way you can encourage them: by calling and listening, an encouraging note, offering a ride, seeing if they want to get together, or giving them a gift card to their favorite coffee place. Finally, put these names on your calendar, to-do list, or whatever means will help you to give to others in this way, and do it! Afterward, you will enjoy the well-being that comes as a fringe-benefit of helping another. "Give, and it will be given to you. A good measure, pressed down, shaken together and running over, will be poured into your lap. For with the measure you use, it will be measured to you." (Luke 6:38)

Personal Reflections and Plans from Chapter Ten

Scriptures to Contemplate

Write your thoughts about how these passages speak to you.
II Corinthians 4:7-12, 16-18

You have struggled with God and with men

and have overcome.

Genesis 32:28

From this time many of his disciples turned back

and no longer followed him.

"You do not want to leave too, do you?"

Jesus asked the Twelve.

Simon Peter answered him, "Lord, to whom shall we go?

You have the words of eternal life.

We believe and know that you are the Holy One of God."

John 6: 66-69

If this is how God treats his friends, no wonder he has

so few of them.

Teresa of Avila

CHAPTER 11

Wrestle with God

A time to tear and a time to mend.
Ecclesiastes 3:7a

October 6, 1998

Sunday morning. I looked around the large semi-circular church sanctuary from my usual seat in back, a position allowing me to stand or exit if needed, and elevated so I could easily see. The service was full - hundreds of people - but scanning the crowd, my gaze lingered occasionally upon one of the select few, one of the dear ones with whom I now found myself locking arms. Ours was a hidden fellowship, unknown by most, a secret society. The Fellowship of the Suffering was an exclusive membership. Most people had no idea of what we were about.

When I was a child, we used to visit my cousins in their small Texas town. We played outdoors for hours, and then at dusk each evening, I would witness a miracle. Tiny twinkling lights appeared out of nowhere, floating silently in the air all around us: the magic of fireflies. Their lights shown most brightly when darkness fell. We caught them sometimes, holding them in glass jars. But neither the blackness of night, nor their imprisonment, could diminish their light. It was as if darkness and difficulty brought out their brightness more vividly. And now, in my adult life, I was witnessing many such shining lights, undimmed by the dark. Fireflies all around, inspiring me, lighting my path.

I've discovered treasures from the past as I've read books by those who learned to shine in their suffering.

These people have become my mentors,
even though I've never met them.
Just a few pages in the morning or evening
can fuel me for the day.
See Appendix 3 for reading recommendations.

There was Bethany, sitting just a few rows ahead with her husband and three young children. Several years before, she had been diagnosed with multiple sclerosis. Her symptoms at first were minimal. Now, there was greater weakness, fatigue, bodily limitation. Today, she and her husband looked tired and down-trodden from the battle, but there was also a radiance, an inner strength. And there was a *knowing* between us, the *knowing* shared by members of our secret society. It transcends age and background and gender. It is shared by those who have suffered deeply, who have wrestled and fought, and been humbled in the fight. And when we meet another member of the Fellowship, we share a common language, characterized in part by what we *don't* have to say amongst ourselves - words required by outsiders. There is a gentle understanding, a soft smile. Words that are bolstering because of their simple, shared truth and understanding.

Jenny was in our Fellowship as well, sitting closer to the front, hat pulled down to cover her hair loss. A double mastectomy was being followed by chemotherapy in her battle against cancer. Jenny was exuberantly singing to God at this moment, a miraculous joy gracing her like a halo. It followed her wherever she went. I was in awe of it, and knew that I didn't possess this quality in such obvious abundance. I wondered if Jenny was closer to heaven than me, and was seeing it more clearly as she drew nearer.

And then my gaze fell upon the wheelchair - up on the front row, in the aisle, as always. Its occupant slumped, though not in defeat. Bob was in an advanced stage of multiple sclerosis, his mobility greatly limited, and in constant pain. Judy, his wife, sat next to him, a dear and radiant soul. I had known them when Bob was in full health, before these past few years had changed their world. We had been together briefly since my recent arrival, and immediately, there was the *knowing*, the unspoken kinship, even though Bob was mostly non-verbal these days. I knew him largely through Judy now. And Judy was, of course, a full member in our Fellowship. "A nightmare" was how she described her existence to me, yet all the while exuding that unearthly peace and light. We had only managed bits of conversation here and there, and had decided to meet this coming week for lunch. I felt guilty now, seeing Bob's debilitated form on the front row. He wouldn't be coming with us to lunch: just getting out on Sundays was a major ordeal. While I was improving, being set free from my prison, Bob's cage was growing smaller. Their world was far, far worse than mine. What would Judy reveal when we got together? How were they doing it? I could tell we both looked forward to those moments of complete honesty, of not needing to appear strong or wise; of simply being who we were at that moment in our journey, and thereby drawing strength for what lay ahead.

Little did I know that the verbal pictures Judy would paint, the poetry she would express without trying to be literary, would stir and haunt and inspire me for many years to come.

———————————

*Have you discovered a Fellowship of the Suffering,
people who have suffered and are encouraging
and meaningful to you?
Many who suffer become embittered. Instead, seek out the
comradery and rejuvenation
that come from those whose choices
have made them better, not bitter.*

———————————

October 7, 1998

She was an enigma. Sitting across the table from me in Sandy's Restaurant, Judy appeared so simple, unassuming, and unconsumed with trivial things. Her beauty ran deep: true, rich and selfless. Talking with her was like entering a cave that outwardly appeared quite normal. But as soon as you got past the external entrance, you sensed something rare and magnificent. Each new passageway and cavern revealed treasures and time-produced formations of depth, wisdom, insight, and character. And yet she was so down-to-earth, so easy to be around, so inviting.

Judy wanted to hear about me first, commenting that I appeared normal and well. I explained that standing, sitting, walking, moving my arms and hands and head - *everything* - produced pain and felt damaging to muscles and tissues, which could take weeks or months to recover. And I told her about some of my inner struggles from these past months. But despite everything, I *was* slowly getting better, which made me quickly want to move away from discussing my situation that seemed so light compared to Judy and Bob's. Tentatively, I asked what life was like for her, for them.

Judy spoke of their painstaking journey of trying various medical and "natural" approaches; of having Bob's dental fillings removed due to possible mercury leakage, a suspected contributor to MS. "He now has a perfect, white set of teeth," she laughed sadly. I knew her meaning: what enjoyment could he derive from them now, in appearance or function? This past year, there had been high hopes when Bob tried a newly-developed medicine. In response, Bob had plummeted downward, losing mobility and bowel control. Judy worked from her home now, where she could continually care for Bob's many needs. She prayed that God would protect her back as she lifted his large form in the bathroom, or in and out of bed, helping him throughout the day. Finances did not permit outside help. Truly it was a living nightmare, as Judy had said. In all this, though, her sunny disposition was somehow still there.

Bob was in constant pain, and unable to read or use the computer, or do anything to relieve the boredom besides listening to tapes or the radio. I knew from experience how uninviting those become. And yet, Judy said he remained sweet and kind, so appreciative of her efforts for him. Her description made me think of an innocent lamb who is led to slaughter, ever-trusting and mild . . . like the Lamb that Bob followed. Judy said that he knew *this whole thing* was to be his service to God, and his job was to remain trusting and believing in him despite everything. Bob knew, as the doctors had told him, that MS does not shorten one's life span. He couldn't hope for that. It only causes greater and greater debilitation and pain through the years. In light of my recent experience, I despaired thinking of what Bob's daily existence must be like, with the future only promising worse.

"One time," Judy said, "I heard a loud THUD in the next room, and found Bob lying on his back on the floor, tears streaming down his cheeks. He had tried to move himself from one position to another. Looking up at me, he said, 'God is good, God loves me, God is totally in control.' Mary, that is the creed of the suffering, to believe and cling to that in the face of everything horrible that is happening to you."

God is good, God loves me, God is totally in control.

The brightness of Bob's light astonishes me, fortifies me. I feel privileged to have caught glimpses of the amazing inner life he lives, resolute and strong, unfueled by the recognition of people, for heaven's eyes alone. I think that, of all the great spiritual women and men who have done enormous works throughout the centuries, no one could be greater than this man, who can steadfastly hold to *that* perspective, throughout years past and years to come of pain and boredom and hopelessness for anything better in *this* life. In heaven, I will marvel and applaud exuberantly when I see his reward.

I embraced Judy warmly at the end of our time together, holding her for a while. We had exchanged so much love during our brief visit, providing sustenance and fortification for the days ahead.

October 8, 1998

I kicked through piles of red and gold leaves - autumn's final artistry. Crunching, crackling, they laughed, trying to rouse me from somber thoughts. These daily walks had become times of reflection, talking to God. Today I was asking yet again how he could allow such horrible things to happen to people he loved. It was completely in his power to heal Bob, and me, and countless others, with a mere word. *Nothing,* it seemed, could make it worth the misery: no "lesson learned", no "greater prize in heaven", no "higher purpose." Serious pain hurt too much. Could anything be worth the price?

I thought of friends in New Zealand, whose newborn baby had died after a terribly difficult pregnancy, after being saturated with the prayers of multitudes. Then there was a friend's church that, in a year's time, had seen a leader's wife murdered, and two of its young ministers die. Everywhere there were stories of great misery. "Are you really even there, God?" I heard myself whisper.

Gently, quietly, I traced my lifelong mental journey: first remembering my early and later years of study, in which I had carefully weighed the evidence both for and against God's existence, examining both historical and logical evidence. I re-examined the historical validation of the Bible, followed by what it had taught me of this wondrous Being, of his love, kindness, and sovereign control over all. In my mind, I saw an old-fashioned scale, with bronze cups on either side to place objects upon for weighing. I was the woman holding it, blindfolded, weighing the evidence impartially. As I weighed the objective evidence in my mind, the scale ruled heavily in God's favor. And then, added to his side was the vast number of miraculous answers to prayer I had experienced, things that were too difficult to explain apart from supernatural intervention. Things that communicated deep love.

There was *so much* evidence that God exists, and that he loves people, and that he is good, and in control. That what the Bible says about him is true.

On the other side of the scale were the miserable circumstances of people. This side declared that either God didn't exist, or if he did, he wasn't powerful enough or didn't care enough to stop it all. The evidence on this side weighed far less than its counterpart. I thought of books I had read, and their insights.

One of my spiritual mentors, Amy Carmichael, lived and wrote during the early 20th century. For the last two decades of her life, she was a bedridden invalid, but continued to live in India, where she remained involved in her lifelong work of helping orphans. She wrote, regarding her illness, "So though through these months *acceptance* has been a word of liberty and victory and peace to me, it has never meant acquiescence in illness...But it did mean *contentment with the unexplained.* Neither Job nor Paul ever knew (so far as we know) why prayer for relief was answered as it was...Hardly a life that goes deep but has tragedy somewhere within it...And who can spare from his soul's hidden history the great words spoken to St. Paul, "My grace is sufficient for thee, for My strength is made perfect in weakness"? Such words lead straight to a land where there is gold, and the gold of that land is good.

"Gold - the word recalls Job's affirmation, 'When He hath tried me I shall come forth as gold'...The Eastern goldsmith sits on the floor by his crucible. For me, at least, it was not hard to know why the Heavenly Refiner had to sit so long. The heart knows its own dross. Blessed be the love that never wearies, never gives up hope that even in such poor metal He may at last see the reflection of His face. 'How do you know when it is purified?' we asked our village goldsmith. 'When I can see my face in it,' he answered." (*Rose From Brier* by Amy Carmichael, Chapter 3)

Contentment with the unexplained. God hasn't given us all the information to solve the age-old, anguishing riddle of suffering.

There are pieces of the puzzle that won't be seen in this life. But either God exists, or he doesn't. And if he does, he is either good and loving, or he isn't. Either everything that happens passes by his approval, or it doesn't. The evidence is overwhelmingly convincing on the former side in each case. _Somehow_ His goodness and love and allowance of suffering, all co-exist. We simply haven't been given all the information in this life to be able to understand.

For outstanding, uncomplicated reading on questions about God's existence and suffering, check out "More Than A Carpenter" or "A Ready Defense" by Josh McDowell, and "When God Doesn't Make Sense" by Dr. James Dobson. All of these are referenced in Appendix 3, and are easily available on bookselling websites.

Maybe it's like trying to explain color to someone who can see only black and white. Words fall short. Maybe only in eternity can we comprehend the full answers to the questions of suffering. Peace came only when I accepted the fact that I will not know the complete answers on this side of heaven.

The choice before me was clear: either trust in him with all my heart, not leaning on my own understanding, or don't. (Proverbs 3:5, 6) A fellow-pilgrim once said that difficulties either lead a person to become *bitter or better.* Without a conscious effort, the former can automatically take over. I knew from experience and observation that bitterness poisons the container in which it is held. And how could I *not* trust this One whom I had enjoyed and loved for so many years, who had showered me with good things all my life. I had richly tasted, drunk deeply, of this rare, exotic, incomparable One.

When Jesus walked the earth, there was a time when many people turned away and stopped following him because of some perplexing things he was teaching. He asked his devoted follower Peter if he, too, was going to turn away. Peter replied, "Lord, to whom shall we go? You have the words that give eternal life. We believe and know that you are the Holy One of God." (John 6:68, 69)

Job's words, after wrestling with suffering's questions, were, "Though He slay me, yet will I trust Him." (Job 13:15) These and others had been down the same mental path as me, and had come to the same conclusion: I don't understand everything, but how can I *not* follow with all that I *do* understand? Jesus himself was the ultimate example, enduring harsh cruelty, allowed by his Father, yet fully trusting him, later to be richly rewarded. Couldn't God have accomplished the same thing through a painless route for his Son? Even Jesus asked, "Father, if you are willing, take this cup from me." (Luke 22:42) But he didn't let this deter him, for he knew the truth.

Jesus "resolutely set out for Jerusalem" (Luke 9:51), knowing where that road would ultimately lead. (Luke 23) I would embrace him, hold tightly to his hand, though it led me down a dangerous and painful path. I would go wholeheartedly, locking arms with Bob, Judy, Bethany, Jenny, and all the others. I knew too much to do anything less.

For Further Thought

Write your responses on the following pages.

For your spiritual health:

Each person is affected differently by suffering. Some do not experience spiritual questioning, while others find this to be a major part of their journey. Don't be afraid to talk honestly with God about your doubts and frustrations. God included passages like Psalm 44 and Lamentations 3 as models for us in dialoguing with him about our uncertainties. In Genesis 32: 22-32, God blesses Jacob for wrestling with him. Read these, and write your thoughts about how they speak to you.

Also, see Appendix 3 for helpful spiritual resources. If you've never begun a personal relationship with God, or aren't sure that your eternal destination is heaven, read the information in Appendix 4 entitled, *How to Know God Personally.*

Personal Reflections and Plans from Chapter Eleven

Scriptures to Contemplate

Write your thoughts about how these passages speak to you.
John 6:67-69; Psalm 131

So do not worry about tomorrow;

for tomorrow will care for itself.

Each day has enough trouble of its own.

Matthew 6:34

By perseverance the snail reached the ark.

Charles Haddon Spurgeon

CHAPTER 12

Keep Your Oxygen Mask On

A time to be silent.
Ecclesiastes 3:7b

October 16, 2000

"I feel like a human jigsaw puzzle, trying to hold all my pieces in place."

As always, Joni listened intently, warmly. She was one of those lifelong friends whose heart is a place of refuge and strength. Oregon was a taste of heaven because of her presence there.

I continued. "One wrong move might topple everything - vertebrae, shoulders, hips, the works."

"Is that really what they say?" Joni was worried.

"Well, if I follow the explanations of some of these chiropractors and massage therapists to their logical conclusions …. yes. They're putting all these parts back into their correct positions, and if I don't move or sit or stand or walk just right - it'll all fall down like dominoes eventually."

We laughed a minute at how ridiculous it seemed.

"Just trying to always move correctly causes such anxiety - *that's* probably what's keeping me from improving faster. And how can I ever go back overseas if I really buy into all this? I'll need their occasional tweaks and adjustments for the rest of my life."

"And yet, haven't you seen some improvement from them, both the ones in Texas and here?"

"Well, that violent back-cracker I saw a few weeks ago - I just feel blessed to have escaped him unharmed. But the others - yes, I've seen some improvement. But I don't know if my improvement would have been the same without them."

We sat for a few moments in the comfortable silence that only very close friends can enjoy. Joni's home was like a garden - bright splashes of color, dainty textures of lace and fabric, warm wood furnishings. Everything was clean, orderly, and beautiful - a sanctuary.

"I think I'm finished with them all for now. The massage therapist from Eugene is going on vacation for a couple of weeks, and I think I'll see how I progress on my own for a while, not looking for a replacement. If I'm going to return to Budapest, I can't count on someone being there to help me. I can't be dependent on outside help."

"Aren't you afraid you'll go downhill without that massage therapist, or someone?"

"Always. It's a hard risk to take, because I don't have time to spare. We're hoping we might be able to return to Hungary at the beginning of January, so the kids can start school at the beginning of the new semester. But like I said, I need to find out now if I really am dependent on being here, on what America offers medically."

We sipped our warm herbal tea for a moment, savoring cinnamon and apple. Outside, brown leaves fluttered on the porch lattice vines. A cold breeze pierced the sunlit air, trying to reach us. It couldn't.

"Oh Mary, I'll miss you so much." Joni had a way of always making me feel like the most important person in the world. "I want you to be able to go back, but I also don't. And Austin - he must miss you terribly. How's he doing over there all by himself?"

"Well, you know he's living with his friend's family. They say he's doing really well - and Joni, on the phone and in letters, it sounds like he's really growing spiritually. He's making significant choices and changes because of his vibrant relationship with God."

"Really?! Like what?"

"Well, he worked hard to organize "See You at the Pole" - a special meeting of prayer around the flagpole for all the students at his high school to start the school year. And people have written or called us, mentioning how Austin is becoming a spiritual leader at his school. I think it's because he's on his own there - he's rallying and rising because he's independent and making his own decisions. Joni, I was lying in bed the other morning and thinking that, if this whole fibromyalgia catastrophe I'm going through was just so that Austin could become spiritually mature and strong, it would all be worth it."

Joni nodded, knowingly. We'd both concluded that accomplishing *that* in our children's lives is so significant, we'd go through almost anything to see it happen. Joni and I had raised our children together - across the miles - from toddlerhood to teens - comparing notes, encouraging, advising, praying. Cliffs and storms on the journey had made us well aware of the ways we could lose them spiritually or emotionally along the way.

"But Austin's kind of discouraged right now, because we had been hoping we could return to Hungary at the end of October. We've just told him that I'm not doing well enough. My lower back is still so painful and unpredictable - and my shoulders aren't great either. I had another few days of depression admitting to myself that I couldn't return yet. And I hate disappointing Austin and John and everyone. Oh Joni, what if I can't ever return? There's nothing here in America that John and I want to do. No ministry or job motivates us here. We still think that God has led us to Hungary, but with all that's happened, we sometimes wonder."

"Mary - just keep doing your best, taking one day at a time. Let God take care of the future." Her gentle voice smoothed the words in like a balm.

And of course, she was right. But I absolutely dreaded the thought of having to live in America, to retire from the "front lines." I would do whatever God wanted, but thoughts of serving Him anywhere but Eastern Europe were unappealing to me. I felt drawn to the people there, with their openness and kind humility, having endured centuries of hardship. But what if I never got well enough to return? Or what if we decided to try it, but my condition deteriorated to the point that we had to move back to the States?

The disappointment and upheaval would be devastating to us all.

I had learned there were no guarantees. Sometimes the path leads straight through "the valley of the shadow of death," but I was learning to say, "I will fear no evil, for you are with me" (Psalm 23:4). *He* would be with me wherever the path led - *that* was my guarantee. God wanted *His presence* to be my joy - not my circumstances. I had a lot to learn, but he was a patient teacher.

In "When God Interrupts," M. Craig Barnes writes to people who are hurting from an unexpected turn of events, living life as they never expected or planned it.
He likens this dilemma to that of Jonah who was headed one way when God completely changed his direction through an encounter with a giant fish.
Barnes invites us to view our situation through this lens.
Ask God for wisdom to see how he wants to use your illness to direct you in new ways. These may be small or huge: new perspectives, character changes, relationship growth, career alterations, or geographical relocation.
Sometimes we limit God by neglecting to consider completely different directions he may have for us.

November 4, 1998

Winter was creeping in. In Oregon, that meant days upon days of cold, grey, rain. But there were joys, like warm wood fires, and signs of Thanksgiving's approach, to be followed by Christmas.

For me, the new season meant switching my daily walk from a park to the nearby mall. I would walk for 45 minutes, winding through large department stores where carpet cushioned my steps, providing needed shock-absorption. I didn't dare to miss a day of walking the full amount for fear of going backwards.

With the new season also came another MRI for me. This was requested by Dr. Mitford in Houston, just to re-check everything. This one was much easier than my previous experience. I wasn't in nearly as much pain or trauma, and it only lasted forty minutes, not two hours. Everything checked out okay, as before. This was followed by a trip to a podiatrist, to make sure my feet weren't contributing to my back problems. They weren't. And then a final check of my neck by one of the specialized chiropractors, like the one in Austin, who adjusted only the uppermost vertebra so that all others could fall into line. That top vertebra was holding up fine.

I was on a slow, steady incline of improvement. My heart vacillated between getting my hopes up, then guarding itself against disappointment. Could I be seeing a light at the end of the tunnel? I was still far from 100 %, but could possibly make it in Budapest if I reached only 80%. Maybe that wasn't too far away.

John and I continued to visit small church "home groups" in the evenings. We had lived overseas for a long time, and were enjoying getting to know the people again. Hundreds of new people had come to the church since we had lived there nine years before. In the small gatherings, we were encouraged with a warm, sincere, and gracious reception. In a couple of cases, the group asked *John* to speak about this past year, as I sat next to him silently. It felt strange, because *I* was the one going through so much, learning unique lessons from God, going where only a select few had journeyed. Perhaps they thought it would embarrass me if they asked me personally about this difficult phase. After John spoke, people would highly praise him, and he *is* an inspiring communicator. But a little voice inside me longed to be heard: "Don't you people know where I've been, what I've been through, what rare insights I've learned at a great cost?" People were funny, so unaware. I often felt lonely, and different from everyone.

November 18, 1998

John called today from Belarus. This country, formerly a part of
the Soviet Union, had recently become part of our Eastern
European area of responsibility. After careful prayer and
consideration, we had decided it would be good for John to go
from November 11 - 23. Some issues existed among our staff and
ministries there that he was uniquely qualified to address. And
John needed to go. It was hard on him to be biding time in the
States, with only loosely-defined work and goals. After all, *his*
hopes and dreams were on the line as well. He was fantastic about
it to me, but I saw the little signs and knew him well. Also, this
trip was a test to see how I could fare on my own, with the kids,
through daily life, because travel would be a big part of John's
work if we returned to Eastern Europe. And overall, things went
well, apart from one upheaval.

Christmas Around the World was to be a glorious evening in
December for our church women and their invited guests. I felt
honored when they asked me to be the main speaker a few weeks
back, to talk about various Christmas traditions and insights from
different countries. Now, though, as I attempted to write the talk,
my arms got sore and stiff after only a short time on the computer.
Writing by hand was still impossible. And I felt engulfed by
tension and dread when I thought of standing - or probably sitting -
in front of hundreds of women. In my normal physical state, I
loved doing this sort of thing. But now, my physical capabilities
were unpredictable. Even holding my notes in front of me to read
for twenty minutes might be a strain. And I had a panicked feeling
that the content I chose for the night might be a letdown, not at all
what the organizers were hoping for. This illness had robbed me of
so much inner confidence and strength.

So why did I still hold on to this - why not just call back and
say "no"? For one thing, the event was now only two weeks away.

How would they find another speaker at such short notice? And I would feel foolish explaining my reasons for backing out. From outward appearances, I seemed so normal to people that they often couldn't conceive of my limitations, nor the psychological consequences. I would feel embarrassed and humiliated if I had to explain in detail my physical incapacities. I also had the hope, the memory, of the great enjoyment this type of thing could be under normal circumstances. I hated to have to give up yet another activity.

With John away, I needed to get someone else's objective input.

Joni spoke plainly when I called her. "Isn't your uppermost goal right now to get well as fast as possible? From what you've told me, the physical challenges that this presents could set you back for weeks, not to mention the stress. Is it worth that risk?" Like so many times before, God used a dear friend to stabilize and support me. Joni's clarity and firmness made me strong, and helped me to do what I needed to do. I had worked myself into turmoil for a few days, especially without John and his anchoring presence. The phone call saying "no" was difficult, but I felt tremendous relief afterward. Relief from pressure that might have thwarted my healing process. And the event organizers were completely understanding. The speaker God provided for the evening was a well-known, successful author. So I wasn't as irreplaceable as I thought. But then, who is?

How are you at arranging your schedule for yourself in ways
that make you feel better? When you feel better,
you will be able to give to those you love.
Like the airlines tell us, "Put your oxygen mask on yourself
first, then you will ensure that you can
put the oxygen mask on another."

At the end of this chapter, write down 10 small things that you can do for yourself that make you feel better. They should be things that can be easily done, like playing an instrument, taking a bubble bath, doing an art or craft, or reading. Put this list of things in a place where you can see it daily, then do one small thing a day to make yourself feel better. Keeping your inner reservoir full can overflow into better health for yourself, and better relationships with others.

November 23, 1998

John returned from Belarus with stories of freezing cold weather and warm interaction with our staff. There were food shortages, and things like eggs were a treasured delicacy, rare and expensive. He'd made a stopover in Budapest, spending time with Austin, who was indeed doing exceptionally well. Everyone in Hungary was anticipating our return. I allowed myself to become hopeful, even excited: I had weathered John's absence well, managing the essentials of children and home.

"I'm afraid to get our hopes up, John, but…. maybe we could look into airline reservations for the end of December."

We still had our original return flight tickets, which we had continually moved back to new departure dates over the months. Each new date had meant a disappointing letdown, but this one seemed more hopeful than the others. Still, I said, "I'll know I'm returning to Budapest when I'm actually on the plane going back."

Could it really happen this time? Tentatively, cautiously, we decided to make the new reservation and move ahead with preparations for our return to Hungary.

November 26, 1998

Thanksgiving Day. A time of fellowship and feasting with friends.

Things were going superbly. Joni, her husband Ron, their three children, and our family all shared a meal, with memories and laughter. Then out of the blue came a sharp, stabbing pain in my lower back that I hadn't felt before. It was so intense that when I walked, it felt like I might collapse.

Sheepishly, I moved around Joni's house, seeing if I could walk it out a bit.

But my thoughts raced: Could I really ever make it in Budapest? Should I run back to the massage therapist, or the gentle chiropractor? No, I decided resolutely. This would be a good time to test if I could make it without outside medical help. I'd wait it out, walk carefully, see what happened. Yes, there was the risk of going even further backwards. But this was my chance to see if I was really ready to make it overseas.

December 1, 1998

Seventeen years ago on this day, I gave birth to my first child, Austin. *Seventeen years*. It was a landmark birthday, and I wasn't with him. Another thing stolen from me by this evil illness.

I sent Austin a special package, with notes he could open every day for a week before his birthday. Each note contained some money, and a memory I had of his life from the past seventeen years. I grieved about our separation, but God took great care of him. Several of his friends at school baked birthday cakes, and everyone made him feel enormously special, making up for our absence. Again, God's people came through overwhelmingly.

Two families from our Oregon church offered to pay Austin's airfare to Portland for Christmas. We were staggered by their generosity, but accepted the offer, feeling humbled yet again.

After Thanksgiving Day my back slowly improved. Each

day the pain was less sharp, until only the normal dull ache remained. I walked as much as I could, and was back to my forty-five minutes soon. So we were still on track with our imminent departure date, which had become December 31. It was scary, exciting, unbelievable. Would it really happen?

For Further Thought

Write your responses to the following.

For your spiritual, emotional, and relational health:

A study by Dr. Robert Emmons at the University of California, Davis showed that gratitude improves emotional and physical health. So to maximize your improvement in every way, form a habit of expressing gratitude. Write down at least ten things for which you are thankful. Some things on your list might be a sunny day, a reliable car, a meal prepared just the way you like it, extra spending money each month. People can go on your list too. The next step is to express gratitude for each item, whether that means a silent "thank you" to God, or gratitude expressed to another in some way.

Personal Reflections and Plans from Chapter Twelve

Scriptures to Contemplate

Write your thoughts about how these passages speak to you.
Philippians 4:4-9; I Thessalonians 5:16-18

Consider it pure joy, my brothers,

whenever you face trials of many kinds,

because you know that the testing of your faith

develops perseverance.

Perseverance must finish its work

so that you may be mature and complete,

not lacking anything.

James 1:2-4

Never, never, never, never give up.

Winston Churchill

CHAPTER 13

Fill Your Reservoir and Keep It Full

A time to speak.
Ecclesiastes 3:7b

December 7, 1998

Six pairs of identical shoes arrived: a very supportive athletic model, the only style I could wear without aggravating muscles. We couldn't get these in Hungary, and I was planning to stay a long time. Forty bottles of varying vitamins were boxed in the bedroom. There were fifteen canisters of health-producing barley powder to drink daily with water. An extra heating pad had been purchased. Five fibromyalgia resource books lay stacked in the corner, ready for packing. A newly-purchased coat hung in the closet, ready to go. It was full-length, with extra-warm lining and a thick hood. Below it on the floor were two pairs of spiked attachments that could be strapped under regular shoes, to prevent slipping on icy walkways. Our supplies were well-stocked, in anticipation of returning to the Hungarian winter.

In addition to this array of goods for my personal health was a variety of food, medicines, and clothing for our family. Boxes were filled up as our money went out. Was I really going to get on that plane this time? If not, there was going to be a lot of disappointment over these financial investments. The stakes were getting higher, along with our hopes. Would they all come crashing down, or would we actually be in Budapest on January 1? Only God knew, and to be honest, His voice was now indistinguishable amidst doubts and desires.

December 20, 1998

I tried to ignore it, hoping it was only a little thing that would go away on its own. But the pain got worse and worse. Were there unseen forces at work, trying to keep us out of Hungary?

This time it wasn't my back, or neck, or muscles. It had begun with a little bothering ache, which was growing sharper…in my *tooth*. Just a few days before Christmas holidays, and eleven days before our departure. Would a dentist even be able to fit me in?

I finally gave in, admitting that I needed dental help. But could I call the one person who might help me at a moment's notice, the one who had assisted us so much already, helping to provide the house we lived in, the car we drove, even Austin's air flight to Oregon for Christmas? Dr. Lawrence had been exceedingly generous. Could I ask him to look at my tooth in the midst of his rushed holiday schedule? I had to.

Roger Lawrence was a kind, gentle dentist from our church, and he didn't hesitate for even a moment when I called him Saturday night.

"Can you meet me in my office Sunday afternoon? It's not open then, but we need to see that tooth as soon as possible, in case we need to fit in further appointments so you can leave on time."

He suspected a cracked tooth, which would mean that a separate lab would become involved, and their schedule might be tight this time of year.

I could have kissed his feet, and laughed at the incredulity of it all. This was getting absurd. What was next? Gall stones? A brain tumor? Just before leaving Texas, I had come down with an insidious case of poison ivy from an unknown source, while the rest of my family remained unscathed. Why was I the target of so many maladies? I was no longer asking questions, just prayerfully taking the next step, which meant meeting Dr. Lawrence in his office on Sunday, intensely grateful.

When difficulties seem overwhelming, instead of asking,
"Why Lord?"
ask "What Lord?" Instead of "Why did this happen to me?
Why would God allow this?" ask "What do you want me to do?
What is the next step? What is it that you want me to learn from
this? What can I do in this situation to glorify you?"
Asking "Why?" can paralyze you, but asking "What?" opens
a channel for God to guide your thoughts.
The confusion settles like dust and clarity can emerge.
Is there something you're overwhelmed about now? Isaiah
30:19, 21 says "How gracious he will be when you cry for help!
As soon as he hears, he will answer you . . . Whether you turn to
the right or to the left, your ears will hear a voice behind you,
saying, 'This is the way; walk in it.'"
Ask God "What?" then trust Him to guide your thinking.

Dec. 21, 1998

I was to receive a crown, not with jewels, but beautiful gold, on
one of my lower back molars.   My tooth was cracked
and the plot thickened: three more appointments with Dr.
Lawrence had to be fit into the next 10 days, which included
Christmas and New Year's holidays. Even then, it all hinged upon
the independent lab's part in rushing the work this time of year. Dr.
Lawrence would do his best, but he wasn't sure if the lab would
comply. There were no alternate flight dates available to Hungary
until late January. All we could do was wait, pray, and hope I
could be crowned before December 31.

173

December 22, 1998

The phone rang at 5:50 a.m. *What now?* It was a phone call from Hungary, from the father of the family Austin was staying with.

A mother's worst fears infested my mind. *Oh please, Lord, no.* I was becoming shell-shocked, bracing for the next blow.

The father spoke anxiously: just three hours before Austin's scheduled flight from Budapest to Portland, he'd discovered his passport was nowhere to be found. Now, several hours after missing that flight, Austin was on his way to the American embassy in Budapest, hoping to be granted a duplicate passport. He had a newly-scheduled flight departing the following day.

I breathed an enormous sigh of relief.

Rolling with the punches was becoming second-nature now. We were living in a constant barrage of the unexpected and the ridiculous. I seemed to be running a race toward the finish line, all the while having stones hurled to knock me out. What would happen next? Each day held some new and strange surprise.

December 25, 1998

Christmas Day. It was so different from one year before, when we'd arrived fresh and untarnished in Budapest, hopes high and doubts low. We could not have foreseen what lay crouching, waiting to pounce in the year ahead.

A foot of untouched snow lay on the ground outside our cozy little Oregon home, stilling and quieting the world, covering its blemishes. It was a perfect "White Christmas." All was calm, all was bright - at least for a day.

Nestled inside, the five of us were all together again, at last. Austin had arrived safely two days before Christmas, five months since I'd seen him last. It seemed like a very long time. He was different, fresh and alive in his independent walk with God, more responsible and mature; and as always, loving and thoughtful.

I was very different too from a year ago. Subdued, I sat in my supportive chair, watching everyone open presents. Before, I would have rushed around, looking at gifts, picking up wrapping paper and ribbons, throwing them away as I checked the cooking turkey, darting in to grab the camera. I couldn't sit still in my former life, always needing to accomplish something, with little time to stop and savor and snuggle. Forced into stillness, I was enjoying the sights and sounds of the dearest people in the world.

The world stopped that Christmas Day. We didn't look ahead or behind. Tomorrow we would move back into action, back into the race, dodging stones. But today we stopped, and treasured, and adored.

———————

"Mary treasured up all these things
and pondered them in her heart" (Luke 2:19).
Do you take time to savor what is good in your life?
Do you notice things of beauty as you go through your day?
Whether it's a simple bird on the branch by your window,
the sunset as you're driving on the freeway,
or the smile on your loved one's face,
take time to treasure and ponder lovely things.
This is part of filling your reservoir to overflowing.
Make it a habit each week: choose a day to go on a "beauty
hunt", proactively looking for beauty throughout a day, or as you
go for a walk, or as you're driving your car.
This kind of exercise will help train you to find and savor
the positive as a way of life.
For more exercises like this, see my book
"Retrain Your Brain for Joy" in Appendix 2.

———————

December 30, 1998

Tomorrow was the day. Was it really going to happen? "I'll know I'm going back when I'm in the airplane, flying," I kept hearing myself say.

The past week had been filled with dental appointments (my crown had been completed two days before), packing (by the family, as I gave instructions from my chair), final visits with people, phone calls, and last-minute shopping. It was hectic for the others, but always the top priority for me remained staying rested, moving carefully, not overdoing.

"Refill your reservoir and keep it full," had been Dr. Mitford's analogy. I wasn't to push, emotionally or physically, depleting reserves. John and the kids were committed to this; their whole lives were at stake as well. It was frustrating: I loved the adrenaline rush, scurrying around, making plans, getting ready, accomplishing things. Instead I moved slowly, paced myself carefully, rested often. Though much improved, I wasn't all that well yet.

So many things were still out of my reach: I couldn't grocery shop alone, unable to lift heavier items, or to load bags into the car. Driving for more than twenty minutes was out: my arms and legs became too sore. Sitting for lengths of time was unpredictable, ranging from forty-five minutes to two hours before I needed a fifteen minute walk to loosen up. Meal preparation was unpredictable: sometimes I could do the whole thing, sometimes my arms hurt too much halfway through. Writing by hand or playing the guitar were still impossible. I was, perhaps, 70-80% "fully functional," and still uncertain whether further progress or digression would occur.

Digression. How would the long flight back affect me? Getting on that plane would be totally an act of faith, walking on water to see if God wanted to hold me up. John and I felt certain that God even wanted us to try. Like three young men long ago had said, as they stepped into the flames of a huge furnace, "...the

God we serve is able to save us, and he will rescue us from your hand, O king. But even if he does not . . . we will not serve your gods" (Daniel 3:17, 18). We were stepping out, trusting him, however he wanted to work.

December 31, 1998

The first leg of our journey took us back through Austin, Texas. We spent the night there, so I could stretch, walk and rest. Everything went smoothly, until we showed up at the airport the following morning, and were delayed for several hours due to "technical difficulties" with our aircraft. Finally, boarding a different flight, the long, overseas segment began.

I remember a blur of movies, meals, walking around the plane, standing in the aisles, jogging lightly in the tiny bathroom, more meals, more walking, movies, jogging, standing, over and over until ... finally... a stopover in Germany for a few hours. We scanned the airport, searching for a place where I could lie down. A piercing pain in my low back had developed, demanding a reclining position. A metal bench had to do. We propped coats and backpacks, but nothing was truly comfortable. Dozing in and out, I finally heard the loudspeaker announce our concluding, one-hour flight into Hungary.

Reluctantly boarding, I found my seat, jiggling and wiggling all the way to Budapest.

One year before, our flight had descended into the foreboding dark and gloom of a late winter afternoon. Today, the early afternoon sun cheered us through the window as we landed. Affectionate friends welcomed us at the airport with hugs and sincere excitement, eager to bring us home. Outside, the air was chilled, but a recent heavy snow had melted away. Driving through dirty streets, my heart sang. Seeing the broken buildings, the dying cars, my thoughts danced in gratitude to God. I was back! I was here! I was home.

Familiar furnishings greeted us warmly in our apartment. But had I really left it so unfinished? Pictures along the floorboards, unhung. Books stacked in the corner. Tattered, dirty carpets waiting for newly-purchased replacements. It didn't matter. I had made it. I was home.

Our soft, comforting bed awaited, complete with a heated blanket and a therapeutic "egg-crate" mattress. It felt like a cloud as I sunk in, covered with blankets by Austin and John, hovering. Then came kisses from Matthew and Alisa, smiles and softness.

Home. Sleep came quickly, deeply, filled with contentment. And dreams. I dared to dream again.

For Further Thought

What does filling your reservoir mean for you, spiritually, emotionally and physically?

I've listed a few things that are helpful from my experience. Check the ones that you'd like to focus on now, and add your own.

- Spend time daily with God, reading the Bible and talking to him.
- Study the Bible in a discussion group with friends.
- Get involved in a church that helps you to grow spiritually.
- Have good talks with close friends regularly.
- Resolve conflicts with your family and establish healthy relationships.
- Go out regularly for fun with family and close friends.
- Keep exercise, good nutrition, and sleep and top priorities.
- Take vitamins and minerals regularly.
- Pace yourself well and don't overdo it.
- Try a new treatment approach when you've reached a plateau in your improvement.
- (Add your ideas here.)

*Personal Reflections and Plans
from Chapter Thirteen*

Scriptures to Contemplate

Write your thoughts about how these passages speak to you.
Ephesians 6:10-18; I Chronicles 29:11, 12

New Seasons Begin

He reached down from on high and took hold of me;

he drew me out of deep waters.

He rescued me from my powerful enemy,

from my foes, who were too strong for me.

They confronted me in the day of my disaster,

but the LORD was my support.

He brought me out into a spacious place;

he rescued me because he delighted in me.

Psalm 18:16-19

Tis a lesson you should heed, Try, try again.

If at first you don't succeed, Try, try again.

William Edward Hickson

EPILOGUE

Journey With God

A time to love and a time to hate.
Ecclesiastes 3:8a

Those first few months were like waking after a long winter's hibernation and discovering that spring had transformed the world. I went from strength to strength.

People were incredibly welcoming, both those I had met briefly, and those my family had come to know in my absence.

"Oh, *you're* the one we've been praying for all these months."

"So you're *Austin's* mother. You have a fantastic son."

"Where have I heard your name… *Mary Henderson.* Oh, are you John's wife?"

Before long, I was grocery-shopping by myself, driving everywhere, playing my guitar a little, speaking at various functions, language-learning, telling Hungarian people about God's love. It seemed like nothing could stop me. Soon I would be 100%, I thought.

Then came June, and a sudden drop downwards. One day, that horrible feeling returned to my shoulders, as if my arms hung from raw nerves out of their sockets. I was scared. *Just rest a few days,* I told myself. Days turned into weeks, then months. I didn't get worse, but those shoulders and arms were slow to heal. In the previous months I had slipped a bit into unhealthy eating, but now quickly self-corrected. By September, I was fully back, moving ahead, even better than before.

Hopes and dreams were becoming a reality, as I ventured more and more into the lives of Hungarian people and our Eastern European co-workers. Helping them and meeting their needs brought tremendous joy. I made trips to Bulgaria, Slovenia, and Russia, but kept a realistic pace. Rest remained a high priority.

Then came January, and another downward plunge, this one worse than before. The calves in my legs became tight, feeling damaged, refusing to heal. My arms and hands followed in this decline. Walking was difficult, and standing impossible. Grocery-shopping became a thing of the past. Driving was limited to 10 minutes. I stayed home more and more, unable to do things, trying to heal.

Invitations had started coming in, offering opportunities I longed to fulfill. Women in Romania, Albania, Poland and Russia, asking if I could come to their countries, speak at various conferences. I had to decline again and again because of my failing health. Once again, my life was being robbed of rich possibilities.

Discouragement and depression began to wrap their cold fingers around my throat. Was this how my life was going to be now? A roller coaster of ups and downs, hope and despair? Before, recovering in America, I always believed that I would just get better and better, until I reached and maintained normalcy. Now, I was seeing a different pattern, a lifetime of being an invalid, stretching far ahead to the horizon: years upon years of frustration and pain. Inwardly, I felt like a fireball, ready to scale the highest mountain or explore the deepest ravine. And yet, I was confined within this body, this cage, always closing in.

And now, as I write this, it's been twenty-four years since I first arrived in Hungary. My physical capabilities have gone up and down over time, and I've fought many battles, coming to terms with all aspects of this unwanted illness and lifestyle.

And in the process, I've often come back to the lessons of that first year. And I remember the fireflies.

I think of Bob, saying, "God loves me, God is good, God is in control."

I think of Bethany and Jenny, soldiering on, shining through each day, within whatever capacity God gives them.

I think of Amy Carmichael, and her *contentment with the unexplained.*

After returning to Hungary, during one of my most difficult downhill stretches, I read further words of Amy's, written from her bed in India during her difficult final years of illness:

"True valor lies, not in what the world calls success, but in the dogged going on when everything in the man says Stop…the refusal of softness…Let us face it now: which is harder, to be well and doing things, or to be ill and bearing things? It was a long time before I saw the comfort that is in that question. Here we may find our opportunity to crucify that cowardly thing, the softness that would sink to things below, self-pity, dullness, selfishness, ungrateful gloom." (Amy Carmichael, *Rose from Brier,* Chapter 11)

It is *far* more difficult to "be ill and bear things"- soldiering on, unselfishly, choosing thankfulness - than "to be well and doing things," as challenging and tiring as those things may be. The latter is widely acknowledged and applauded; the former is often seen only by God, yet is priceless in value if done for him.

Each day brings opportunities, large and small, to make secret choices for God's eyes alone: attitudes and thoughts, along with their resulting words and actions. Though no one sees these choices or knows how difficult they are, there is great reward in them. And there is a hidden garden, full of rare and unearthly pleasure, in learning to rejoice when no one besides God sees these choices.

But my life these past twenty-four years has not required deprivation from outside activity. Far from it! For five years, I continued working beside John, serving over 1000 staff throughout 18 countries. People traveled to us in Budapest, and I would occasionally travel to them. I'm thankful we live in the century where phones and computers have revolutionized communication possibilities. And my children grew up strong in this journey. I see God's smile in their shining eyes.

After five years living in Hungary, my condition plummeted to an all-time low in late 2002. I returned to the States, where we are now living. I've tapped into resources and treatments that have returned my health to the best it's been since this entire journey began, and I've attained a remarkable level of wellness. I now live a normal, active life. In fact, friends say that I'm a miracle. I love my life here in the States, doing things that bring the deep joy and fulfillment that come when you know you're where God designed you to be.

Life is an unfinished jigsaw puzzle with several pieces missing. I wish this account could end with all the pieces in place, a picture of perfect clarity. But perfection is for the next life, not this one, and the Craftsman will complete everything then. Perhaps God will complete the fibromyalgia section of the puzzle with my body becoming completely symptom-free on this side of heaven. I'm doing all within my power to bring that about.

But whatever happens, I know where the Light is found, the Source of radiance and tranquility. And if I lose my way, I'll look for smaller twinkling lights, shining in darkness, sometimes in jars, brightening the path until the fullness of Day.

Personal Reflections and Plans

Go back through the pages at the end of each chapter, and re-read your proposed goals and plans. Record here the next steps you plan to take in order to accomplish each goal, and refer to the resources listed in the appendices for additional information.

Scriptures to Contemplate

Write your thoughts about how this passage applies to you.
Psalm 18

A Note from the Author

My experience with fibromyalgia, of winding through an uncertain maze of medical options, is not unique. Most people with chronic illness have experienced frustration and despair, along with discovery, in trying to find things that will help them. In the following pages, I have included some suggested resources to help fellow sojourners on this path.

Along with resources for physical health, I've also provided information for those seeking emotional and spiritual fortification. Growth and development in these areas is important for everyone, but especially for those facing significant challenges in the physical realm. God bless you on your journey!

Mary Henderson

Appendix 1

Helpful Resources for Chronic Illness

As I mentioned in Chapter 4, a helpful treatment philosophy for my chronic illness was presented by one of my doctors, an MD who utilizes many integrative/alternative treatments along with conventional medicine. This approach works well for a broad range of illnesses. He said that he'd seen hundreds of patients with chronic illness, and for each one of them, it was a different combination of treatments that brought improvement. What worked well for one person may not have any effect on another. The approach he recommended, therefore, was to work through a list of treatments that have worked well for many patients with your illness, and discover which ones cause you to improve.

Following this philosophy, I've seen dramatic improvement in my symptoms. I've used a combination of conventional and integrative/alternative medicine, but it's mostly the latter that works for me and most other fibromyalgia patients I've known. The things that have helped me the most are massage therapy; eating nutritionally and eliminating simple carbohydrates; acupuncture; chiropractic; various detoxification treatments; vitamin and mineral supplements; thorough testing and ongoing treatment for food and environmental allergies; and a general philosophy of eliminating everything toxic from my life and adding healthy choices.

The bottom line for everyone with a chronic illness is this: get your body as healthy as possible. We don't have the luxury of cutting corners with nutrition, exercise, toxins, etc. Get your physical body to its absolute healthiest, and maintain that. Your other symptoms may decrease, perhaps drastically, as a result, and you will decrease your chances of adding another, perhaps worse, illness as you grow older.

The following are some helpful resources that may guide you in your pursuit of optimum health. Many of these include extensive listings of alternative health resources:

1. Frahm Health Solutions

David J. Frahm is a naturopath, nutritionist, and master herbalist who offers a comprehensive approach to long-term illness utilizing alternative approaches that have been highly effective for many. He has written several books, including one containing a detailed plan for proactively battling illness, *A Cancer Battle Plan Sourcebook* (publication details listed below). Many have found the first version of this book to be the most helpful. Mr. Frahm explains and evaluates a number of common alternative health treatment options. He is located in Colorado, but does health consultations via phone. His email address is dfrahm6873@aol.com. For further details, see his website at https://www.frahmhealthsolutions.com

Frahm, David J. 2000. *A Cancer Battle Plan Sourcebook.* New York: Jeremy P. Tarcher/Putnam

2. Jordan S. Rubin battled his way to health from severe chronic illness. His book, *The Maker's Diet,* offers a variety of helpful information regarding alternative approaches. Rubin has earned degrees in naturopathic medicine, nutrition, and natural therapies. He's written numerous books and has appeared on over 300 TV and radio programs worldwide.

Rubin, Jordan S. 2004. *The Maker's Diet.* Lake Mary, Florida: Siloam, A Strang Company.

3. A comprehensive book on fibromyalgia is *Fibromyalgia and Chronic Myofascial Pain Syndrome, A Survival Manual, 2nd Edition* by Devon Starlanyl, MD and Mary Ellen Copeland, MS, MA. This book's appendices contain extensive lists of resources which can benefit all chronic illness patients. Dr. Starlanyl's

website is also very informative: https://fmcmpd.org/index.htm

Starlanyl, Devon and Copeland, Mary Ellen. *Fibromyalgia and Chronic Myofascial Pain Syndrome, A Survival Manual.* 2nd Edition, 2001. Oakland, CA: New Harbinger Publications, Inc.

Appendix 2

Resources for Emotional Growth and Encouragement

1. As part of my training to become a licensed counselor, I learned the practices and principles of *mindfulness,* which can be very helpful with illness and pain. Mindfulness is defined as *learning to live in the present moment nonjudgmentally.* Mindfulness involves relaxation and visualization exercises that calm your body and mind, and train your brain to focus on your current moment peacefully. This results in greater well-being physically, as well as mentally and emotionally. Scientists have discovered that mindfulness techniques help improve physical health in a number of ways: it helps to relieve stress, treats heart disease, lowers blood pressure, reduces chronic pain, improves sleep, and alleviates gastrointestinal difficulties, along with other things. As a start, check out my book about this and an app that I find helpful:

Henderson, Mary. *Rest for Your Soul: Practice the Present. Practice the Presence.* 2021, USA. On amazon.com

My Life is an app with mindfulness exercises that are about three to ten minutes long. These help train your brain to live in the current moment, to lower anxiety, and to improve your physical and mental well-being. You can find it in your App Store. It has a picture of a smiling cloud on the icon.

MyLife, Inc. Version 7.35. *My Life App.* https://my.life

2. *Retrain Your Brain for Joy* is my book about experiencing joy. Wherever you are on your wellness journey, whether facing minimal or major obstacles, you can train your brain to experience greater joy and fulfillment. When living with illness, it's vital to continually focus on the positive, on the portion of your glass that is "full." *Retrain your brain for joy* contains 31 little exercises that

help you to do exactly that. As you start through this book, it will be like playing a game throughout your day, creating a secret inner life that increases your well-being. Along the way, you're transforming your mindset and creating new lifelong habits.

Henderson, Mary. *Retrain your brain for joy: 31 Mini-Adventures.* 2021. Amazon.com

3. The following are two nationwide organizations that can connect you with a Christian counselor:

Focus on the Family's website contains a number of valuable resources on a variety of subjects, including chronic illness. This organization also has a nationwide network of counselors, that can be accessed through their website or by phone. http://www.focusonthefamily.com/ (Scroll to the bottom of the page to "Find a Counselor") 1-800-A-FAMILY

New Life Ministries is another source for locating a counselor. Their website also contains helpful resources including several online groups for interacting about specific issues such as depression, boundaries, and fear and anxiety. http://newlife.com 1-800-NEW-LIFE

Appendix 3

Resources for Spiritual Growth and Encouragement

1. Barnes, M. Craig. *When God Interrupts: Finding New Life Through Unwanted Change*. 1996. Downer's Grove, Illiois: InterVarsity Press.

2. Brother Lawrence. *The Practice of the Presence of God*. 1958. Grand Rapids, MI: Spire Books.

3. Carmichael, Amy. *Rose from Brier*. 1972. Christian Literature Crusade.

4. Dobson. James. *When God Doesn't Make Sense*. 1997. Wheaton, Illinois: Tyndale House Publishers.

5. Dunn, Ron. *When Heaven Is Silent*. 2008. CLC Publications.

6. Elliott, Elizabeth. *A Path Through Suffering: Discovering the Relationship Between God's Mercy and Our Pain*. 1992. Vine Books.

7. McDowell, Josh. *A Ready Defense*. 1993. Nashville, Tennessee: Thomas Nelson, Inc.

8. McDowell, Josh. *More Than A Carpenter*. 1977. Wheaton, Illinois: Tyndale House Publishers.

Appendix 4

How to Know God Personally

What does it take to begin a relationship with God? Do you earn his favor by devoting yourself to unselfish religious deeds? Become a better person so that God will accept you? Live by a strong moral code? None of these is the basis for entering into a relationship with him. God has made it very clear in the Bible how we can know him. Let me explain how you can personally begin a relationship with God right now...

1. First of all, know that God loves you and created you to know him personally.

God created you. Not only that, he loves you so much that he wants you to know him now and spend eternity with him. Jesus said, *"For God so loved the world that he gave his only Son so that everyone who believes in him will not perish but have eternal life."1*

Jesus came so that each of us could know and understand God in a personal way. Jesus alone can bring meaning and purpose to life.

So, what keeps us from knowing God?

2. Secondly, all of us sin and our sin has separated us from God.

We sense that separation, that distance from God because of our sin. The Bible tells us that *"All of us like sheep have gone astray; each of us has turned to his own way."2*

Deep down, our attitude may be one of either active rebellion or passive indifference toward God and his ways, but it's all evidence of what the Bible calls sin.

The result of sin in our lives is death: spiritual separation from God. 3 Although we may try to get close to God through our own effort, we inevitably fail.

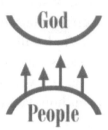

This diagram shows the great gap that exists between us and God. The arrows illustrate how we might try to reach God through our own efforts. We may try to do good things in life, or earn God's acceptance through a good life or a moral philosophy. But our good efforts are insufficient to cover up our sin.

How then can we bridge this gulf?…

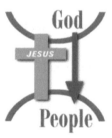

3. My third point is that Jesus Christ is God's only provision for our sin. Through him we can know and experience God's love and plan for our life.

We deserve to pay for our own sin. The problem is, the payment is death. So that we would not have to die separated from God, out of his love for us, Jesus Christ died in our place. On the cross, Jesus took all of our sins on himself and completely, fully paid for it. *"For Christ also died for sins...the just for the unjust, so that he might bring us to God."* 4 *"...he saved us, not because of righteous things we had done, but because of his mercy."* 5

Because of Jesus' death on the cross, our sin doesn't have to separate us from God any longer. *"For God so loved the world that he gave his only Son, so that everyone who believes in him will not perish but have eternal life."* 6

Jesus not only died for our sins, he rose from the dead. 7 When he did this, he proved beyond doubt that he can rightfully promise eternal life - that he is the Son of God and the only means by which we can know God. That's why Jesus said, *"I am the way, the truth and the life; no one can come to the Father except through me."* 8

Instead of trying harder to reach God, he tells us how we can begin a relationship with him right now. Jesus says, *"Come to me." "If anyone thirsts, let him come to me and drink. Whoever believes in me... out of his heart will flow rivers of living water."* 9 It was Jesus' love for us that caused him to endure the cross. And now he invites us to come to him, that we might begin a personal relationship with God.

Just knowing what Jesus has done for us and what he is offering us is not enough. To have a relationship with God, we need to welcome him into our life…

4. The fourth and final principle is that we each must individually accept Jesus Christ as our Savior and Lord. The Bible says, *"Yet to all who received him, to those who believed in his name, he gave the right to become children of God."*10

We accept Jesus by faith. The Bible says, *"God saved you by his special favor when you believed. And you can't take credit for this; it is a gift from God. Salvation is not a reward for the good things we have done, so none of us can boast about it."* 11

Accepting Jesus means believing that Jesus is the Son of God, who he claimed to be, then inviting him to guide and direct our lives. 12 Jesus said, *"I came that you might have life, and have it more abundantly."* 13

And here is Jesus' invitation. He said, *"I'm standing at the door and I'm knocking. If anyone hears my voice and opens the door, I will come in."* 14

How will you respond to God's invitation?

You can begin a personal relationship with God by receiving Christ right now. Remember that Jesus says, *"I'm standing at the door and I'm knocking. If anyone hears my voice and opens the door, I will come in."* 15 Would you like to respond to his invitation? Here's how.

The precise words you use to commit yourself to God are not important. He knows the intentions of your heart. If you are unsure of what to pray, this might help you put it into words:

Jesus, I want to know you. I want you to come into my life. Thank you for dying on the cross for my sins so that I could be fully accepted by you. Only you can give me the power to change and become the person you created me to be. Thank you for forgiving me and giving me eternal life with God. I give my life to you. Please make me the kind of person You want me to be. Amen.

If you sincerely asked Jesus into your life just now, then he has come into your life as he promised. You have begun a personal relationship with God. What follows is a lifelong journey of change and growth as you get to know God better through Bible reading, prayer and interaction with other Christians.

The following are verses I referred to above:

(1) John 3:16
(2) Isaiah 53:6
(3) Romans 6:23
(4) 1 Peter 3:18
(5) Titus 3:5
(6) John 3:16
(7) 1 Corinthians 15:3-6
(8) John 14:6
(9) John 7:37,38
(10) John 1:12
(11)Ephesians 2:8,9
(12)John 3:1-8
(13)John 10:10
(14)Revelation3:20
(15)Revelation 3:20

Appendix 5

Leading a *Breaking Free* Discussion Group

Whether your group consists of 2 or 20 people, the following guidelines will be helpful in leading your group effectively.

Each member of the group can read one or two chapters per week, and write their responses to the questions and verses in the text and at the end of the chapter. They can also underline thoughts in the chapters that are particularly meaningful or helpful to them.

Begin your meeting with prayer, then lead the group through the questions and verses, inviting members to share their thoughts freely. Don't forget to include questions that are within each chapter, as well as at the end.

Ask group members to discuss any portions that they underlined in the chapters.

End your time by praying as a group for each person, particularly praying regarding what each shared in terms of struggles or goals. Don't forget to thank God for the good things happening in group members' lives, and to praise God for various aspects of who He is.

About the Author

Born in Florida, Mary Henderson moved with her parents and sister to Colorado, North Dakota, Wyoming, and Louisiana. She completed her undergraduate degree at the University of Texas in Austin, and her masters degree at Hope International University in Fullerton, California. In a career that has spanned more than 40 years in Christian ministry, Mary and her husband John have lived and worked throughout New Zealand, Eastern Europe, Russia, and the United States. Mary currently divides her time between counseling, writing, speaking, theater, and her family. She and her husband have three grown children.

Mary has written two other books:

Rest for Your Soul: Practice the Present. Practice the Presence
Retrain your brain for joy: 31 Mini-Adventures

Both are available on amazon.com.

For more information about Mary Henderson and her books, visit http://www.maryhenderson.org

Made in United States
Troutdale, OR
10/17/2024

23868363R10141